LOVING SOMEONE
WITH A MENTAL ILLNESS OR
HISTORY OF TRAUMA

LOVING SOMEONE
with a
MENTAL ILLNESS
or
HISTORY OF TRAUMA

Skills, Hope, and Strength for Your Journey

MICHELLE D. SHERMAN, PhD, ABPP
AND DE ANNE M. SHERMAN

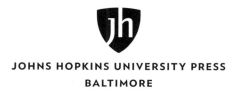

JOHNS HOPKINS UNIVERSITY PRESS
BALTIMORE

© 2025 Michelle D. Sherman and DeAnne M. Sherman
All rights reserved. Published 2025
Printed in the United States of America on acid-free paper
Illustrations by James Monroe Design

9 8 7 6 5 4 3 2 1

Johns Hopkins University Press
2715 North Charles Street
Baltimore, Maryland 21218
www.press.jhu.edu

Library of Congress Cataloging-in-Publication Data

Names: Sherman, Michelle D., author. | Sherman, DeAnne M., author.
Title: Loving someone with a mental illness or history of trauma : skills, hope, and strength
    for your journey / Michelle D. Sherman and DeAnne M. Sherman.
Description: Baltimore : Johns Hopkins University Press, 2025. | Includes bibliographical
    references and index.
Identifiers: LCCN 2024010628 | ISBN 9781421450506 (paperback) | ISBN 9781421450513
    (ebook)
Subjects: LCSH: Mentally ill—Family relationships. | Psychic trauma—Patients—Family
relationships. | Families of the mentally ill.
Classification: LCC RC455.4.F3 S467 2024 | DDC 616.89—dc23/eng/20240613
LC record available at https://lccn.loc.gov/2024010628

Special discounts are available for bulk purchases of this book. For more information,
please contact Special Sales at specialsales@jh.edu.

CONTENTS

WELCOME

If you love someone with a mental illness or history of trauma, this book is for you. Welcome. We know this can be a challenging and demanding role. When your loved one is doing well, you may feel calm and hopeful; however, watching them struggle can be immensely painful. Your personal journey may parallel their unpredictable ups and downs. You may dedicate a lot of time and energy to supporting your loved one, and it can be easy to neglect your own feelings and needs.

The fact that you picked up this book reflects your commitment to yourself. Welcome. Dedicating this time will hopefully yield benefits for you as well as for your relationship with your loved one.

Is This Book for You?

This book is for family members and friends who care about an adult who has a mental illness or has experienced trauma. We specifically address major depression, bipolar disorder, anxiety, schizophrenia, and post-traumatic stress disorder (PTSD). For ease of reading, throughout this book we generally use the term "mental illness" to encompass a wide range of mental health disorders.

Although mental health conditions have specific symptoms and each person's experience of mental illness is unique, many of the feelings and challenges faced by family members and friends are similar. For example, consider a mother whose daughter cuts off communication when seriously depressed, and a wife whose husband's PTSD leads him to be emotionally withdrawn and anxious at family activities. Although the histories and diagnoses differ, both of these women may feel lonely, hurt, worried, or sad; they might struggle with how to communicate and connect with their loved one; and they may be unsure how to respond to others' questions about their loved one's well-being.

What Can You Gain from This Book?

Although many valuable books explain various aspects of mental illness, we wrote this book for you as the family member or friend . . . providing hope and strength for *your journey.* It's important for you to be seen and to have your experience validated.

We do not strive to provide all the answers; easy solutions simply don't exist for complicated situations. However, we do offer a great deal of research-based information, empowering and practical skills, up-to-date resources, and optional interactive activities to guide you in reflecting on your feelings and experiences. Specifically, you will

- Learn tools to cope with difficult emotions

- Reflect on strategies to empower your loved one, including when navigating the complex mental health care system

- Acquire skills for strengthening your relationship with your loved one

- Learn effective communication and limit-setting skills

- Consider how stigma and discrimination around mental illness have affected you and your loved one

- Learn strategies to support your children and help them cope effectively

- Explore ways of managing common challenges, such as when your loved one declines professional help or misuses alcohol or drugs

- Understand how your loved one's traumatic experience can impact you and your relationship, and how the two of you can work together as a team

- Find ways to build your personal resilience and be compassionate with yourself

How Can You Get the Most from This Book?

You don't need to read the entire book or go through the chapters in order. Instead, check out what applies to your situation and take what speaks to you.

Throughout the following chapters, we offer opportunities to reflect on your thoughts and feelings, including open-ended questions, interactive activities, and checklists. We invite you to grab a pen or pencil and dive in.

Writing can provide a chance to name, organize, and process your experiences. Spelling and grammar don't matter, so please jot down whatever arises in your heart, mind, and spirit. Of course, all of the exercises are optional, but we encourage you to give them a try.

There are many well-documented benefits of writing from the heart. For example, writing about deeply personal emotions and thoughts can decrease blood pressure, strengthen your immune system, decrease depression and anxiety, and improve sleep and overall well-being.[1] Writing can also give you the opportunity to find deeper meaning in the challenges you are facing and perhaps understand your situation from a new perspective.

Be thoughtful about where you keep this book after you have added your reflections. It's important to feel safe to write without censoring or worrying that others may read it. If you prefer, or if this book is not your personal copy, you could record your responses in a private journal or notebook or in digital form.

If you start to feel overwhelmed at any time, please take a break and draw upon your own support network and professional team. Come back if and when you wish. If a specific section is hard, perhaps skip to the next chapter, or check out the list of Activities to Lift Your Spirit (appendix B). As you work through the book, take what works for you. You are in control. This is your process, and this book is meant to support you at your own pace.

By the way, if you don't like writing, consider expressing yourself in another way that works for you—paint, draw, create poetry, make music, and so on.

Why Did We Write This Book?

Suffering in silence can magnify confusion, isolation, and pain. We wrote this book so those who love someone living with a mental illness or history of trauma can be comforted, validated, educated, and empowered. As a daughter–mother, psychologist–teacher team, we ground this book in both our personal lived experiences and in Michelle's 30+ years of clinical experience working with individuals, couples, and families who live with a variety of mental illnesses.

Michelle, a board-certified clinical psychologist, has committed her career to working with families in which an adult has a mental illness or PTSD. Thus, she has been privileged to be welcomed into the lives of thousands of families managing a mental illness, and has a first-hand perspective of their journeys. She has not only gained intellectual understanding of the family experience of mental illness, but also has developed tremendous respect, empathy, and appreciation for their journeys. She brings this academic knowledge and open-hearted sensitivity to creating this book. The information and recommendations herein are grounded in research, in self-compassion principles, and in the evidence-based therapy models of cognitive behavioral therapy (CBT) and acceptance and commitment therapy (ACT).

In Michelle's work across diverse settings, including as a professor in two medical schools and director of the Family Mental Health Program in a VA Medical Center, she has been repeatedly struck by how many family members and friends feel invisible. They frequently work tirelessly to support their loved one, but their experience and efforts are often ignored. Inspired by this awareness and desiring to help, Michelle created family education programs regarding mental illness and PTSD in the late 1990s. In personally facilitating these group sessions, Michelle was in awe of what transpired among these family members and friends, including the power of connection, the ability to be understood, and the knowledge that they are not alone. Group participants were often hungry to learn new skills and to both give and receive support from other families. Michelle wanted to try to emulate and translate some of this experience into a book format, so she approached her mother (and coauthor of books for teens) about joining her in the writing process. This book is the result of this 30-year journey and reflects our commitment to seeing and supporting people like you.

DeAnne is a lifelong educator who has taught a wide range of students in diverse settings. As an advocate for mental health, she volunteers with the National Alliance on Mental Illness (NAMI)–Minnesota, writes self-help books with her daughter, and copresents workshops about mental illness in the family.

Equally importantly in our writing process of this book, we drew upon our own lived experiences as we journey with beloved family members and friends who have a mental illness or have experienced trauma. Our lived experiences inform every angle of our work; they highlight the considerable gap in the available resources, ignite and sustain our passion, motivate us to produce the best possible work, and make our writing especially meaningful.

In the pages that follow, we balance straightforward, research-based information and recommendations with an empathic voice to attempt to connect with both minds and hearts. We strive to create a space in which you can move beyond simply learning facts to courageously and honestly looking at your experience. In addition to presenting strategies grounded in science, we offer recommendations and tools that have helped other families, as well as quotes from family members and friends who have generously shared their stories and allowed us to use their own words.

We hope this book will offer comfort, guidance, strength, and useful skills for your journey.

Michelle and De Anne

Note

Some mental illnesses have unique family impacts that are not addressed explicitly in this book, such as autism, eating disorders, obsessive compulsive disorder, personality disorders, and serious substance use disorders. Although we hope that the content of this book will be useful, we encourage you to seek disorder-specific resources as well. Furthermore, we do not address issues related to parenting children under the age of 18 who have emotional or behavioral challenges; you might check out the NAMI's Basics educational program for that type of support (www.nami.org).

This book is not intended to be a substitute for professional help. If you or your loved one has thoughts of wanting to hurt themselves or someone else, seek emergency care immediately. You can contact a trained crisis counselor via the Suicide and Crisis Lifeline at 988 (call or text) or use their website for chat services: www.suicidepreventionlifeline. org. If anyone is in immediate danger, call 911.

GUIDE TO USING THIS BOOK

As noted in the Welcome, you don't have to read the entire book or read the chapters in order. This guide can help you decide what sections would be most useful to you.

IF YOU ARE	CHECK OUT
Feeling a lot of worry, sadness, anger, exhaustion, or guilt	**Chapter 1** helps you reflect on your experience of these emotions
Struggling with how to cope with intense emotions	**Chapter 2** describes many effective coping tools **Appendix A** lists emotion words to help you reflect on your feelings **Appendix B** describes activities to lift your spirit
Unsure what to tell other people—how to balance your loved one's wishes with your need for support	**Chapter 3** explores considering your loved one's wishes while also seeking support for yourself
Encountering stigma and discrimination in people who do not understand mental illness	**Chapter 4** explains stigma and discrimination and offers tools for addressing it with family members and friends
Missing how your loved one used to be . . . or feeling sad about how the future has changed	**Chapter 5** helps you reflect on the losses you and your loved one may be experiencing

IF YOU ARE	CHECK OUT
Asking yourself what you could have done—and what you could do—to help your loved one . . . and feeling powerless	**Chapter 5** describes six tips for moving toward a mindset of acceptance
Unsure what to say to empower and comfort your loved one	**Chapter 6** lists over twenty encouraging messages.
Uncertain how to motivate your loved one	**Chapter 6** explores how to empower your loved one to set and work toward goals and to foster meaningful relationships.
Unsure how to find reputable treatment services or how to evaluate their quality	**Chapter 7** describes tools for locating mental health professionals and screening questions to ask potential providers
Wondering how you can work effectively with your loved one's health care team	**Chapter 7** provides tips on how to interact with health care providers, including regular communication and dealing with privacy laws
Wanting to strengthen your connection with your loved one	**Chapter 8** offers tips on how to express your fondness for your loved one, as well as ideas for enjoying quality time together
Frustrated by not feeling heard by your loved one . . . or worried and hurt when they shut down	**Chapter 9** reviews helpful communication tips, both for sharing and for responding
Wanting to set limits and respond to challenging situations in a respectful manner	**Chapter 10** describes a four-step process (4Cs) for handling triggering issues
Worried about how conflicts with your loved one can spiral out of control	**Chapter 10** teaches a Time Out process for taking a break from escalating arguments
Wanting to grow the intimacy and connection in your relationship with your intimate partner	**Chapter 11** offers tools for strengthening the bond in your intimate relationship

IF YOU ARE	CHECK OUT
Concerned about the impacts of mental illness or trauma on your children and not sure what to tell them	**Chapter 12** includes eight ways to help your kids understand and cope with parental mental illness and the effects of trauma
Pleading with your loved one to get help for their mental illness	**Chapter 13** explores how to deal with times when your loved one declines help
Struggling with the consequences of your loved one's alcohol or drug misuse	**Chapter 14** explores the role of substance misuse among people managing a mental illness
Wanting to be compassionate about your loved one's traumatic experience(s) and know how to best support them	**Chapter 15** describes common reactions to trauma, as well as how survivors and families can be affected. Tips on how to provide support surrounding trauma-related symptoms are offered
Managing frequent crises, such as hospital admissions, self-harm, suicidal behavior, or violence	**Chapter 16** offers guidance on dealing with mental health emergencies, including identifying warning signs and creating a crisis plan
Wanting to reflect on your own well-being and consider setting a goal to improve yourself	**Appendix C** is a self-assessment that invites you consider several domains of your life
Curious about getting involved in formal efforts to combat stigma and discrimination	**Appendix D** describes several organizations that share a mission of ending stigma and discrimination around mental illness
Wondering what types of mental health services might be helpful for your loved one and for yourself	**Appendix E and F** list many treatment options for people with a mental illness and those that love them
Feeling very alone . . . like no one can understand your experience	**Appendix F** lists support groups where you can connect with others with similar experiences

SNAPSHOT
OF YOUR STORY

To begin, we offer you an opportunity to take a few minutes to reflect on your current situation. The following questions guide you in creating a snapshot of how things are going for you and your loved one—both areas that are going well and issues you are struggling with.

About Your Loved One

What are three things you admire or appreciate about your loved one? _____
_____
_____

What brings your loved one pleasure or happiness? _____
_____
_____

What helps your loved one feel good about themselves? What gives them a sense of meaning and purpose? _____
_____
_____

What goals is your loved one working toward? _____
_____
_____

What is your loved one struggling with right now? What are their biggest challenges or sources of stress? _____

_____

_____

Thinking about your loved one, circle the number that you think reflects their

Current overall level of well-being:

1	2	3	4	5	6	7
Really Struggling			*OK*			*Very Good*

Level of involvement with mental health care:

1	2	3	4	5	6	7
Not at All			*Some*			*Active*

Connections with other people:

1	2	3	4	5	6	7
Very Isolated			*Some Connections*			*Very Connected*

About You

What are three strengths that serve you well in supporting your loved one? _____

_____

_____

_____

What sustains you when your energy or spirits are low? _____

_____

_____

What gives you hope? _____

_____

_____

What is the most difficult part of your loved one's situation for you right now?

_____

_____

_____

Circle the number that reflects your

Current overall level of well-being:

1	2	3	4	5	6	7
Really Struggling			*OK*			*Very Good*

Understanding of your loved one's illness:

1	2	3	4	5	6	7
Very Little			*Some*			*Very Good*

Connections with other people:

1	2	3	4	5	6	7
Very Isolated			*Some Connections*			*Very Connected*

Perhaps your answers to these questions are part of your motivation for picking up this book. We hope that reading the chapters ahead will prove beneficial in many of these domains. If you find this kind of reflection to be useful, you may enjoy doing the more detailed self-assessment in appendix C.

Part I

REFLECTING ON YOUR EXPERIENCE

Chapter 1

YOUR EMOTIONAL JOURNEY

L OVING SOMEONE WITH A MENTAL ILLNESS can feel like a rollercoaster ride. Because your loved one may experience a lot of ups and downs, it makes sense that you might have a wide range of feelings as well.

Although sometimes you may feel alone and believe no one can understand what you're going through, your experience is shared by many. In fact, about 1 in 4 American adults experiences any mental illness, and approximately 1 in 20 adults experiences a serious mental illness (bipolar disorder, major depressive disorder, schizophrenia, or schizoaffective disorder) every year.[2] You are definitely not alone.

IN THIS CHAPTER, YOU WILL

✓ Explore feelings of
  o Worry and anxiety
  o Sadness
  o Anger (and how to deal with unsupportive people)
  o Guilt
  o Exhaustion
  o Hope

✓ Consider a self-assessment of your overall well-being

Coping effectively with strong feelings begins with *naming* and *accepting* them. Both of these tasks can be difficult.

"Only when we can access our feelings, sit with them, name them, and make sense of them, can we ever learn to manage them."

—JULIE MENNANO[3]

As you reflect on your emotions, please be gentle with yourself. Rather than judging yourself or evaluating your feelings as "right" or "wrong" or "good" or "bad," try to remember that they are part of your unique experience. Instead of listening to your nagging internal critic, name your emotion and give yourself permission to feel whatever it is you feel at the moment . . . such as, "I'm feeling pretty sad and frustrated right now." You don't need to rush to fix, deny, analyze, understand, change, or run away from your feeling. For starters, just name it, and allow yourself to be present with that emotion. You may find the list of feeling words in appendix A to be useful.

Remember: Having feelings is part of what makes us human. Emotions can give us information, energy, insight, connections to other people, and motivation to act. Although the *behaviors* we choose based on strong feelings can have consequences, the feelings themselves aren't inherently good or bad. They just are part of your experience. The more you lean into accepting your feelings without judgment, the less frightening and overwhelming they become, and the more you can manage them effectively.

This chapter offers opportunities to consider your experience of several emotions commonly experienced by people who love someone with a mental illness. Then, chapter 2 explores healthy ways of coping with strong feelings.

Worry and Anxiety

When we worry, we ruminate on what could go wrong in a specific situation, such as if you might fail a test or lose a job. Worrying about a loved one with a mental illness is almost universal among family members and friends.

What worries you most about your loved one? What questions or thoughts pop up regularly for you?

EXAMPLES:

- *Who will take care of my adult son when I'm no longer able to?*

- *Will my mom be able to handle the stress if she returns to work?*

- *How will we afford all these doctor bills? Insurance only covers so much . . .*

- *What if my daughter goes back to drugs to escape her depression?*

- *What will happen if my dad stops taking his medication? I know he hates the side effects of weight gain and headaches, but I just worry . . .*

- _____

"I don't know what to do when my son cuts me off and is unreachable . . . it's a constant fear that something bad is about to happen."

—A MOM

In addition to worrying, you may experience more general anxiety, which is not focused on a specific situation. Anxiety can be more diffuse feelings of dread and fear, such as never knowing when you might get an upsetting phone call. In addition to worrisome thoughts, you may find it hard to concentrate and tend to be forgetful. Sleep can be especially difficult when your mind races with fear, doubt, and "what if" questions. Many people experience anxiety physically, such as sweating, chest pain, exhaustion, and headaches. You may struggle to relax and feel "revved up" much of the time. Anxiety may feel like a nagging queasiness in your stomach, or it might involve full-blown panic attacks.

Think about your experience of anxiety. What do you notice in your

Emotions _____

Thinking patterns _____

Body _____

Three aspects of mental illness understandably contribute to anxiety and worry. First, **mental illness often goes in cycles, and the unpredictability can be hard.** Your loved one may do well for a long period but then go through a rough phase. Sometimes the cause of the difficult period is clear, such as losing housing, facing an anniversary of a traumatic event, discontinuing medications, or going through a divorce. Other times, the reason is a mystery. Because of these ups and downs, you may worry a lot about your loved one, wondering if and when another tough period might occur.

A second challenging aspect of mental illness is that **many symptoms are not visible,** and there are no blood tests that offer concrete data on emotional well-being. For many physical health problems, symptoms are visible and lab work can shed light on one's health status. Even just taking someone's temperature at home can give you useful information. This objective data can guide treatment and help you understand what's going on. In contrast, the science of understanding physical markers of mental health problems is in its infancy, and there's no simple thermometer or lab test for mental illness.

Third, mental illness can be especially stressful due to its **ambiguity.** Behaviors that could be due to mental illness can have many causes. For example, you're worried because your daughter is spending a lot of time in bed: is she having another episode of depression? Or is she having migraine headaches again? Or is she just worn out after a demanding semester at college and wants to re-charge? How can you know? In addition, due to the very nature of mental illness, sometimes people struggle to assess their own well-being, and they may choose to keep their struggles to themselves. Lacking objective medical data and being unsure how much your loved one is telling you can understandably leave you feeling anxious and worried.

A Note about Adult Children and Siblings

Parents who have adult children living with a mental illness may experience unique challenges. Although parents generally anticipate their kids will leave home in their late teens or early twenties, people with a serious mental illness may benefit from lifelong support. As a parent, you may worry about your child's ability to be safe, to be financially stable and able to manage their money, to enjoy close relationships, to have meaningful activities, and to have safe housing. At the same time, your possibly lifelong caregiving responsibilities may limit your personal freedom and dreams. It's common to feel resentful at the sacrifices you make.

When worried about your loved one, you may understandably dedicate a great deal of time and energy to them. This can result in other family members, including children, getting less of your support. They may feel ignored and left out and may grow to resent the person with the mental illness. Therefore, you may make an effort to spend quality time with other family members and talk about a variety of topics, not just your loved one.

Furthermore, with age, parents often grapple with questions of who will care for their child when they are no longer able to. Other relatives, especially siblings and adult children, may be called on to play greater roles in caregiving, which can be consuming and overwhelming. Mental health professionals and lawyers can assist families in planning and navigating these situations. Even with open communication and planning however, worrying about your adult child and their future is extremely common.

Sadness

Watching your loved one struggle with a mental illness can be incredibly sad. Sometimes you may have a passing disappointment or a tear comes to your eye, while other times your heart feels like it's about to break. The pain can be overwhelming.

What aspects of your loved one's journey are especially sad?

EXAMPLES:

- *I feel heartbroken every time my wife is admitted to the psychiatric unit. Explaining to our kids why Mommy isn't coming home is so hard . . .*

- *My son's total isolation is hardest for me. All of his friends have ghosted him.*

- *It's hard to watch my boyfriend struggle to do even little things when he's depressed. Just getting out of bed and taking a shower seem like monumental tasks. I hurt for him.*

- *I feel sad when I see my daughter get tense and anxious at the fireworks on the 4th of July; the loud sounds bring back vivid memories of her combat experiences in Iraq. My heart just aches seeing her struggle.*

- _____

> "Why does my brother have to have bipolar disorder? It's just not fair. Sometimes I look at his friends from high school who seem to have such 'normal' lives and wonder why he has to deal with this. My feelings spiral all over the map— sad, angry, confused, powerless. I know it's a real burden for our parents, too, and I hate to see them hurting . . ."
>
> —A SISTER

Sadness can manifest itself in many ways, such as physical sensations of heaviness, a weight on your shoulders, a burden, or even chronic pain. Sadness can also show up in your thinking patterns, such as forgetfulness, difficulty concentrating, or intense pessimism. You may also find yourself isolating from others, being more irritable, crying often, or having less patience than usual. It may be hard to empathize with people whose problems seem insignificant compared to what you're managing.

One way to think about sadness surrounding mental illness is to consider the losses both you and your loved one have experienced. Chapter 5 describes several aspects of grief that you may relate to, as well as some tools in moving toward acceptance of the losses.

> "The most difficult part for me was seeing how it (schizo-affective disorder) changed my son's life. One moment he was a typical kid going off to college and the next he is in a psych ward with a disability. Seeing him in torment and not being able to fix it is horrible."
>
> —A DAD

Take a moment to check in with yourself. Write five words to describe what sadness feels like for you: _____

_____

_____

Anger

The emotion of anger sometimes gets a bad reputation, as if somehow it's wrong or bad to feel angry. Some people deny or avoid the feeling, which can make matters worse. Anger is a normal, even healthy emotion that can give important information. It can also motivate us to set limits, make changes, and advocate for what is right.

Remember: It's important to separate the *feeling* of anger from how people *behave* when they're angry; expressing any feeling in aggressive, abusive ways is never OK.

Think about your experience of anger. What do you notice in your

Body (such as sweating or clenching your jaw) _____

_____

_____

Thinking patterns (such as racing thoughts or difficulty concentrating) _____

_____

_____

Behavior (such as raising your voice or making threats) _____

_____

_____

If you've gotten irritated, annoyed, or downright livid, know that such feelings are common and understandable in light of the often stressful journey of loving someone with a mental illness. In this section, we consider your anger from two angles—first your feelings toward your loved one and then your feelings toward other people.

If you're experiencing anger toward yourself, that is often reflecting guilt, which is addressed next.

ANGER TOWARD YOUR LOVED ONE

Anger toward your loved one can be tricky. Sometimes you might hesitate to allow yourself to feel irritated with them . . . after all, they have a mental illness. However, feeling angry is perfectly normal.

Everyone we care about can make decisions that upset us. We may feel disappointed in their choices, worry about their well-being, and feel angry when they act in hurtful ways. That's part of close relationships.

When dealing with your loved one with a mental illness, you probably have many similar reactions and feelings, but the situation can be more complex. You may ask yourself

- *How much of their behavior is due to their mental illness?*

- *Am I asking too much? Are my expectations unreasonable?*

- *How do I balance having empathy with holding them responsible for their behavior?*

- *Does my loved one understand how their behavior impacts me?*

- *Why doesn't my loved one seem to appreciate all I do for them?*

. . . All are challenging questions with no easy answers.

> "I never thought she (my wife living with bipolar disorder) appreciated how hard it was for me to become the caregiver while doing my best to keep up at work and sacrificing other things and relationships in my life."
>
> **IZZY GONCALES**[4]

You may also wonder if your loved one intentionally uses their mental illness as an excuse for certain behaviors (such as, "After all, I have bipolar disorder, so I can't . . ."). This may feel manipulative and frustrating. It may be hard to know when and how to hold them accountable. Talking to their mental health providers can provide insights into how to handle these tricky situations.

In addition, you may feel especially angry when your loved one (a) declines professional help; (b) engages in dangerous behavior such as substance misuse, violence to others, self-harm, or suicidal behavior; or (c) is unable to recognize or understand their illness (termed *anosognosia*—discussed in chapter 13). These situations are addressed in part III of this book.

As anger is such an important topic, we address how to manage it in your relationship later in this book, including chapters 9 (Communication) and 10 (Limit Setting).

What does your loved one do (or not do) that is especially frustrating for you?

EXAMPLES:

- *I'm so angry that my husband didn't go to our daughter's dance recital. That seems so selfish . . . he felt well enough to go out to the bar but not to the recital?*

- *I'm so frustrated that my daughter continues to smoke in the house when we've asked her to go outside or use the garage.*

- *I'm furious my partner went gambling and lost $5,000 when she was in a manic phase; we had planned to use that money for a family vacation.*

- *I hate when my son goes back to smoking pot. It messes with his antipsychotic medication, and the voices get more intense.*

- *I cannot stand when my partner is sweet and energetic with her friends but then comes home and collapses on the couch. She hardly even talks to me. It's like she puts on this facade in public but then has no energy for me . . . it's just not fair.*

- _____

  _____

  _____

ANGER TOWARD OTHERS

In addition to feeling angry with your loved one, you may experience irritation and frustration with other people in your life. You may have little tolerance for people who make judgmental, uninformed, or stigmatizing comments about mental illness or your loved one. You may want to protect your loved one from such judgment and criticism. You might resent and feel jealous of other families that appear to be immune to the challenges associated with mental illness.

Consider the following diagram that shows Laura's anger in dealing with her dad who has bipolar disorder. She wrote about angry feelings and thoughts toward her family members and friends, her God or Higher Power, and her dad's doctors.

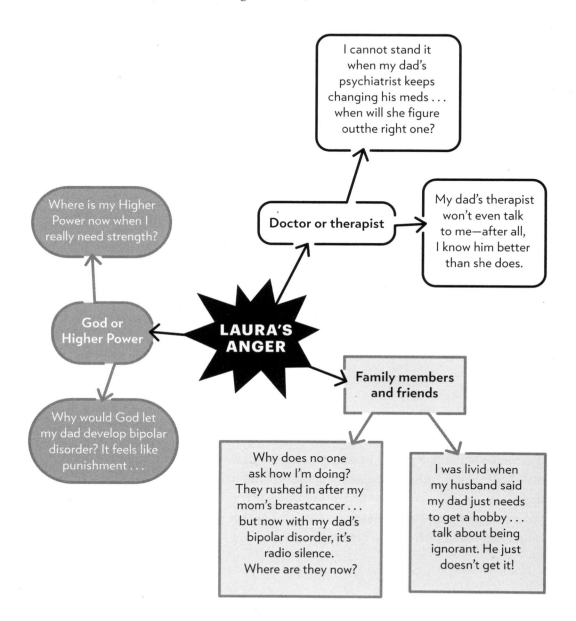

Now fill in this diagram to describe your experience of anger. Write the source of your anger in the blank designs that emanate from "My Anger," and then describe your thoughts and feelings in the remaining designs.

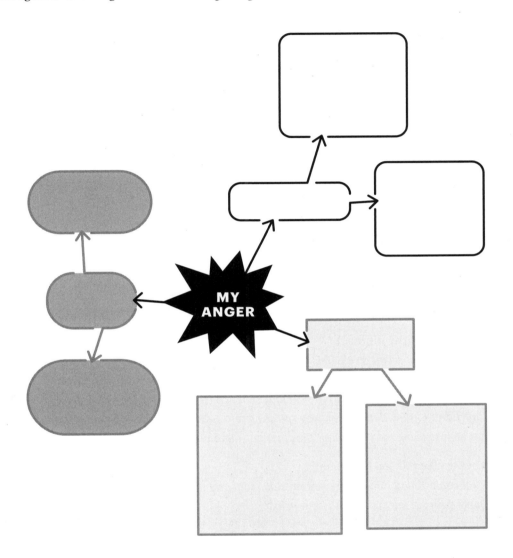

A Note about Dealing with Unsupportive People

Figuring out how to deal with people who dismiss, minimize, or ridicule mental illness or your loved one is incredibly difficult. Although some people don't understand mental illness and have no idea what you're going through, they offer advice anyway. Such unsolicited feedback, while likely well intended, can be hurtful, and you may feel like saying "If you only knew . . . ."

You may try to educate unsupportive people about mental illness and how it impacts families. You can give them suggestions on how to be supportive. However, changed attitudes and behavior toward you or your loved one may or may not follow.

These situations can be trying and frustrating and can affect your relationships more broadly. Ultimately, it's helpful to focus on what you have control over. Protect your energy and pick your battles. You may decide to distance yourself from judgmental people. Setting such limits may be painful. Reach out to people who you can count on to offer compassion, understanding, and hope.

Guilt

Guilt can show up in many ways when someone you love has a mental illness. When you wrestle with questions like "What should I have done?" or "What did I do wrong?", you're likely experiencing guilt.

Consider the following common sources of guilt among family members and friends:

- Wondering if you caused the illness
  - *Was I a bad Mom?*
  - *I hate to see my daughter struggle with depression just like I do—did I cause it?*

- Missing signs of the illness
  - *Looking back, it seems so obvious that my wife was depressed when she distanced from all of us. She put on such a happy mask . . . how did I miss it? My heart just aches thinking of how hard it must have been for her to hide so much from us.*
  - *Why didn't I know that my son was spiraling into such a dark place? I now understand that he was using meth to escape his pain, but I had no idea . . .*

- Not being able to keep them safe
  - *What could I have done to prevent my dad from attempting suicide? I check on him every couple days . . . but can only do so much.*

- Being unable to convince them to get treatment
  - *Why didn't my brother go back to rehab? I'm so sad that he relapsed and got another DWI.*

- Believing you are responsible for their behavior and well-being
  - *If only I hadn't nagged him about cleaning up his office, maybe he wouldn't have blown up like that at the kids.*

- Taking time for myself and my own happiness
  - *I feel so guilty and selfish when I go out with my friends. I need time away, but I hate leaving him alone just staring at the TV.*

"How do you enjoy your own life when your loved one is suffering? It took me years before I left my husband in charge of our son and went on vacation with a friend—just to relax."

—A MOM

If you relate to some of these feelings, consider responding to these prompts:

If only I had _____

If only I hadn't _____

I regret _____

I wish I would have _____

Why didn't I _____

Reflecting on guilt can be difficult, so please remember to focus on all the ways that you *do* show up for your loved one:

Even when I question or get down on myself, I know I do a lot that makes a real difference. I feel good about how I support my loved one in these ways: _____

_____

_____

_____

Guilt can arise in other ways as well. You may feel guilty for having certain emotions or reactions. For example: "*I shouldn't be impatient and short with him. After all, he lives with so much anxiety*" or "*I know she's doing the best she can . . . I really shouldn't feel disappointed.*"

Have you ever found yourself feeling guilty for having certain emotions? ___Yes ___No

If so, what messages did you give yourself? _____

_____

_____

How might you give yourself permission to make space for all kinds of feelings—without judging them? What new, honest message could you give yourself? _____

_____

_____

Feeling guilty about certain emotions and reactions is common, but please remember that all of your feelings are understandable. It's not helpful to berate yourself. Instead, give yourself permission to experience all of your feelings, just as they are.

A NOTE ABOUT MANAGING GUILT

Carefully examining guilt can remind us of our ultimate powerlessness. At the end of the day, no matter how much we care, try, plead, beg, and advocate, our loved one makes their own choices. Admitting and accepting our powerlessness over their behavior can be challenging and sometimes a lifelong process.

If you have regrets, are you ready to let go of some of them? Might you acknowledge that you were doing your best? No one else can do this work for you; it's an inside job. Releasing guilt is a process, not a one-time event, so you may work on this bit by bit over time.

Sometimes a ritual can be helpful in releasing your guilt. You may write your thoughts and feelings down and then rip up or carefully burn the paper, or you might share your writing with a therapist or member of the clergy.

> "As an engineer by training, I want to fix things . . .
> I know I can't just fix her depression . . . letting go
> of trying to change her is the hardest part of the job."
>
> —A HUSBAND

If you're experiencing feelings of guilt, might you be ready to release some of its hold on you . . . and let it go (perhaps even partially)? If so, what could you release?

_____

_____

If now is not the time, that's OK . . . how would you know when you are ready?

_____

_____

It's OK:
- ✓ To make mistakes
- ✓ To not be perfect
- ✓ To put my own needs first
- ✓ To have regrets
- ✓ To disappoint my partner
- ✓ To feel angry with him
- ✓ To say no
- ✓ To take time for myself

—A WIFE

Exhaustion

Supporting someone with a mental illness can be exhausting, especially when your loved one is going through a particularly tough time.

Beyond the emotional demands of supporting your loved one, you may spend a lot of time advocating for them within complex systems such as insurance companies, the health care system, disability offices, and the legal system. The financial aspects of mental illness can also be stressful. Because treatments and medications can be expensive, family members sometimes take on additional jobs to manage the costs, which can contribute to the fatigue.

You may experience exhaustion in your mind, body, and spirit. Cognitively, you may have difficulty concentrating and making decisions; you may also be more forgetful than usual. Your body may feel run down, and any pre-existing physical pain or health problems may flare. Chronic fatigue can also increase the chance of becoming physically ill. Emotionally, you may feel overwhelmed and drained. You may find yourself more irritable and pessimistic than usual, and it may be hard to be motivated to complete everyday tasks.

It's not surprising that exhaustion can manifest in other parts of your life as well. For example, you might miss work more often, or perhaps your performance isn't up to your typical standard. You may also feel so tired that you don't have the energy you normally do for your relationships. You may withdraw or be less present for others in your life.

REMEMBER

- Exhaustion is real.

- Taking care of yourself is imperative.

- Think of the journey as a marathon, not a sprint. Pace yourself over time.

- Ask for help.

- Regular physical activity is one of the best ways to sustain your spirit and energy.

- Remember to breathe, eat regularly, and rest.

Enough said.

> "The most challenging part is unpredictability. Just when things seem to be going well, there can be very real, unexpected setbacks. The path to healing and wholeness is seldom smooth and steady. That can be exhausting."
>
> —A DAUGHTER

> "When my daughter is in crisis, I feel more tired than when I had a new baby for the first time—much more tired . . ."
>
> —A MOM

Hope

Hope can be a tricky emotion when loving someone with a mental illness. On the one hand, there really are many reasons to be hopeful:

- Many people living with a mental illness improve,[5] which may include
  - Full remission
  - Considerable reduction in symptoms
  - Using healthy coping skills to manage symptoms and minimize their impact on everyday life

- New treatments are being developed, including medications, psychotherapies, peer services, community outreach services, and more

- Researchers continue to study many aspects of trauma and mental illness, such as
  - Causes and risk factors of different illnesses
  - Factors that bolster resilience and recovery
  - Prevention and early intervention strategies for at-risk individuals

- Recognizing that mental health is more than just managing symptoms, the treatment field is embracing a recovery model (discussed in more detail in chapter 6) which focuses on
  - Broader wellness, overall quality of life, and access to stable housing and meaningful employment
  - Meaning and purpose in life, including how one spends their time, develops relationships, and works toward goals
  - Collaborative doctor–patient relationships that capitalize on people's strengths. This can involve making treatment decisions together, engaging family members in care, using a trauma-informed and culturally responsive approach, and incorporating peer support

Take a moment to think about your loved one. Describe a time when you felt hopeful.

EXAMPLES:

- *My best friend finally got on a medication that seems to be helping.*

- *My stepson just started a job that will get him out of his room and around other people— I hope it will lift his mood.*

- *We finally have a psychiatrist who communicates with the entire family; she listens to all of us and values our perspectives.*

- *I'm so relieved my fiancé started the DBT (dialectical behavioral therapy) program. Even though it's a long drive from our rural town to the clinic, I've heard such good things. I hope she will learn some helpful skills to help manage her strong feelings.*

- _____

"I was proud and hopeful when my wife finished drug court and got a job. We were on top of the world."

—A WIFE

> "It gives me hope that they are developing new treatments for mental illness all the time. If one does not work for my stepson, we try another."
>
> —A STEPMOM

> "My wife toughed through TMS (transcranial magnetic stimulation) and ECT (electroconvulsive therapy). The fact that she persevered gave me hope."
>
> —A HUSBAND

On the other hand, we acknowledge that it can be hard to hold onto hope, especially if your loved one has recurring, severe difficult spells or crises. Perhaps you've seen periods of stability in the past, only to be disappointed when your loved one discontinues their medication or therapy or makes choices that exacerbate their symptoms. We honor that watching your loved one go through these ups and downs can make it difficult to stay hopeful.

> "I've been hopeful many times, but it's paralyzing . . . I'm afraid to be disappointed again."
>
> —A WIFE

Has there been a time when it's been hard to be hopeful? If so, what was that like for you?_____

_____

_____

As we will discuss in chapter 5, part of the journey of acceptance is realizing you have limited control over the course of your loved one's illness. You can work to prepare for the future, but strive to stay in the present, be optimistic, feel grateful for everyday blessings, draw upon your faith or spiritual belief system, use humor, and stay connected to your support system.

As you've read through this chapter, perhaps other feelings have arisen as well. Use this space to write about them if you wish:

Self-Assessment of Your Own Well-Being

In this chapter, you have reflected on your experience of several common emotions. When caring about your loved one, it's easy to lose yourself. You're so busy and exhausted that you don't take the time to check in on your own well-being. However, you cannot fully show up for your loved one if you don't take care of yourself.

We encourage you to consider doing a self-assessment of how things are going right now in multiple domains of your life. See appendix C, Self-Assessment of Overall Well-being, for a reflection activity.

Perhaps in reading this chapter or completing the self-assessment, you realize or are reminded of your own level of distress. If you are struggling right now, remember you are not alone. As noted at the beginning of this chapter, about one in four adults experiences a mental illness every year[1]—and you're dealing with a painful situation with no simple solutions. Researchers have documented that people who love someone managing a serious mental illness are themselves at elevated risk for some physical and psychological problems, such as insomnia, headaches, fatigue, and depression.[6]

If you find yourself unable to perform everyday activities or are overwhelmed by your distress, please reach out for help. You might start with confiding in a trusted family member or friend or seeking professional help. The next chapter in this book will introduce you to many helpful coping tools as well.

Because the heartache surrounding loving someone with a mental illness can feel devastating, there may be times that you might want to escape the stress and emotional pain. If you have thoughts of wanting to die or harm yourself, please reach out immediately. Any time night or day you can go to the emergency room or call or text **988**, the Suicide and Crisis Lifeline.

You may also try to escape by engaging in potentially addictive behavior to numb the pain, such as gambling, exercising excessively, or drinking more alcohol than is healthy for you. Although these may distract you temporarily, they generally aren't helpful in the long-run. We encourage you to be mindful of risky habits.

The appendices at the end of this book include many resources and ways to find help. If you find yourself in crisis or trying to cope in ways that aren't working, don't wait! Help is available.

Chapter 2

YOUR COPING TOOLS

NOW THAT WE HAVE EXPLORED several common emotions among people who love someone living with a mental illness or history of trauma, this chapter offers skills for managing difficult times. We will review your existing coping tools as well as some new strategies you might wish to try.

IN THIS CHAPTER, YOU WILL

✓ Consider your loved one's behaviors that are most difficult for you

✓ Read stories that portray healthy coping tools

✓ Reflect on your current coping tools and ones you may want to try in the future

Dealing with Behaviors That Are Difficult for You

Some of your loved one's behaviors may just be irritating, and you can simply ignore them. Other things can be upsetting over time, and you find yourself running out of patience. Some behavior can be frightening, and you may feel afraid or just not know what to do.

My Loved One's Behaviors That Are Challenging for Me

Consider the following list of symptoms and behaviors that are common among people with a mental illness. Check those that you see in your loved one now.

Difficulties with Mood or Anxiety

- Being especially down, sad, or hopeless
- Crying frequently
- Low energy and motivation
- Mood swings
- Showing very little or no emotion, or seeming indifferent
- High levels of worry, fear, or anxiety attacks
- Restlessness, inability to relax, or hyperactivity

Concerning Behavior

- Sleeping too much or too little
- Eating large amounts of food or not eating enough
- Not bathing, showering, or changing clothes regularly
- Stopping previously enjoyed activities
- Spending large amounts of money
- Not keeping up with everyday responsibilities such as paying bills, chores, homework, cleaning, work
- Spending extreme amounts of time on social media, video games, or the internet
- Drinking to excess, misusing prescription medications, or using drugs
- Discontinuing medications or therapy

Dangerous, Violent, or Risky Behavior

- Actual or threatened violence toward property, pets, or people
- Self-injury, such as cutting
- Talking about wanting to die or end their life, or attempting to do so
- Driving in an unsafe manner
- Driving while under the influence of alcohol or drugs
- Aggressive behavior during nightmares

Changes in How They Interact with You

- Spending a lot of time alone
- Talking too much or being unwilling to talk
- Being aloof, numb, or emotionally unavailable
- Being demanding and impatient
- Irritability or angry outbursts
- Change in interest in physical intimacy including sex

Issues Often Related to Psychosis

- Seeing things other people do not see
- Expressing beliefs that aren't held by most people in one's culture (delusions), such as having special powers
- Hearing voices, including those saying to hurt themselves or other people
- Being suspicious or seeming paranoid
- Appearing confused or struggling to think clearly
- Acting in peculiar ways
- Talking to themselves

My Loved One's Behaviors That Are Challenging for Me, continued

Looking at the behaviors you checked, think about how they impact you (the list of feelings in appendix A may be helpful).

Behavior _____ How it affects me _____
_____
_____

Behavior _____ How it affects me _____
_____
_____

Behavior _____ How it affects me _____
_____
_____

Your reaction may depend on how you're feeling at the time. Some days a certain behavior may bring you to tears, while other days you take the situation in stride. Remember that you are doing the best you can in a very difficult situation.

Coping Tools

You have probably developed your own strategies for dealing with your loved one's mental illness, some of which work better than others. There are many ways to get through difficult times, and appendix B (Activities to Lift Your Spirit) lists activities you might want to consider.

The following nine stories depict family members and friends using a variety of coping tools, namely strategies for dealing with challenging feelings and difficult life situations. All of the approaches in these stories have been shown to be helpful in managing stress and improving well-being. As you read this chapter, ask yourself what strategies you might consider and how you could fit them into your schedule. Incorporating self-care into your routine can help you stay committed to keeping your own needs a priority.

There are no quick fixes for hard situations, and what is helpful for one person may not work for someone else. You also may want to try a new coping tool several times to see if it helps. Let's consider the following strategies.

Connect with a Support Group

Mariana's daughter was recently diagnosed with major depression. While hearing this diagnosis was difficult, it helped Mariana understand her daughter's worrisome behaviors—spending most of her time in bed, crying a lot, cutting off contact with her friends, and missing a lot of work.

Mariana had gone through a period of depression herself in her 20s, so she recognized some of these behaviors. She always worried that her daughter might experience depression someday as well, so seeing this was heartbreaking.

Mariana read online about a support group for parents, so she tried it out. In the group, she felt comfortable talking to other families who understood what she was going through. She learned about how to support her daughter and ways to take care of herself as a mom. Hearing other families talk about their experiences reminded Mariana that she was not alone. It made a huge difference.

Participation in support groups and educational programs can provide an invaluable opportunity to connect with others who can relate to your experience. For example, participants in the National Alliance on Mental Illness (NAMI) Family-to-Family class have reported numerous positive outcomes, including a greater sense of empowerment, decreased anxiety, and improved abilities to cope and engage in self-care.[7] Chapter 3 explains many wonderful programs provided by NAMI; details on many other classes and support groups for family members of adults managing a mental illness are listed in appendix F.

Be Physically Active

Shalonda spends a lot of time helping her husband manage his bipolar disorder, including reminding him about his medications and scheduling doctor appointments. She feels pulled in so many directions and struggles to make time for herself.

She manages stress by doing yoga classes on Saturday mornings and walking the treadmill in their apartment twice a week. Even when life feels overwhelming, the endorphin rush and peace of mind she gets from exercising keep her committed to these routines.

Physical activity can come in many forms and is one of the best things you can do for your physical and mental health. Although national guidelines recommend adults get at least 150 minutes per week of moderate-intensity aerobic activity every week,[8] doing some amount of exercise is better than none. Even just 11 minutes of moderately intense activity per day is associated with significant health benefits.[9] Also, it's well documented that physical activity is highly effective for improving symptoms of anxiety and depression, with some studies showing its impact to be similar to that of psychotherapy and medications.[10] Physical activity in nature may have additional benefits for mood and energy, so walking at a local park might magnify the impact.[11]

Make Time for Yourself

Noah's sister has schizoaffective disorder, an illness that includes both symptoms of schizophrenia and mood symptoms such as depression or mania. She lives in a group home. He visits her twice a week and talks regularly with her social worker.

Noah relaxes by regularly playing pool with his friends and taking his golden retriever to the dog park. He also keeps a regular sleep routine as he knows he needs rest to be present for his sister. Taking time to recharge with these regular activities and prioritizing his sleep keep him grounded and able to be the kind of brother he wants to be.

Taking time for yourself can enable you to gain a new perspective, refuel your energy, and focus on your own needs. Failure to commit time for yourself can leave you emotionally depleted, physically exhausted, and potentially resentful of your loved one. One often-neglected yet very important part of taking care of yourself pertains to sleep. Getting sufficient rest is vital for your physical and mental health and can help you cope with the stress of supporting your loved one.

Try Meditation and Deep Breathing

Mei lives with her parents, her husband, and their three kids. Her dad experiences paralyzing anxiety and frequent panic attacks; he doesn't leave the house very often. He is a very proud man, deeply grounded in his traditional Chinese culture. Because he sees mental illness as a weakness, he feels ashamed about his anxiety and tries to hide it from his family.

Mei maintains her well-being by practicing mindfulness meditation and recently started using an app on her phone. She practices square breathing and enjoys listening to music. Taking that time to center herself gives her more patience and empathy in supporting her dad.

Note: Square breathing is an especially helpful technique that is explained on page 122.

Mindfulness and meditation can have benefits for mental health, and some specific approaches such as mindfulness-based stress reduction have well documented positive impacts.[12] Similarly, deep breathing can quiet your nervous system, thereby calming your mind, helping you relax, and improving your ability to manage stress.

Distract Yourself

Danielle and Yumi are college seniors and best friends, having lived together for four years. While Danielle is excited about graduation, Yumi worries about the future and doesn't know what she wants to do. She has shut down, quit going to class and doing homework, and spends most of her time in bed; she smokes marijuana and drinks three or four glasses of wine most days.

Although Danielle works hard to help Yumi feel better, trying to be her cheerleader can feel overwhelming and discouraging. To keep her own spirits up, Danielle regularly goes to movies with friends and hangs out with her boyfriend. She also goes to her folks' house and plays with their new puppy, Luca, the best cuddler ever. After getting off campus and distracting herself, Danielle is rejuvenated and has more energy to be a good friend to Yumi.

Intentionally shifting your attention away from emotional pain or stress temporarily can be healthy. Distraction allows you to get some distance from the situation, and your feelings may be less intense when you return. You may feel more energized, optimistic, and confident in your ability to handle the stress after having taken the break. Distraction is different from avoidance, as the intent here is to return to the situation later.

Strive for Acceptance

Enrique's son became addicted to opiates after taking prescribed pain medication following knee surgery. Although his son had dealt with panic attacks before blowing out his knee, the pain and inability to return to his construction job made the anxiety a lot worse. Although Enrique tried to convince his son to get professional help, it just wasn't happening.

Enrique heard about the 3Cs at an Al-Anon meeting (a peer support group for adults who care about someone managing an addiction): *I didn't Cause it, I can't Cure it, and I can't Control it.* Although this saying originally referred to loving someone who misused alcohol or drugs, it also applies to mental illness. As Enrique embraced this concept, he was able to accept his son where he was and stop trying to change or fix him. It wasn't easy and required a lot of support from his friends, but it made a big difference in his well-being and, ultimately, in his relationship with his son.

Working toward acceptance allows you to release efforts to change a situation or someone else, thereby surrendering your attempts to control, judge, or fix. It's saying: *"Yes, this is the reality . . . it's painful . . . I can't change it or them . . . and I choose to accept it . . ."* Although accepting difficult situations and feelings can be challenging and may require repeated decisions, it is a skill that can be learned (see more in chapter 5). Leaning into a mindset of acceptance can be freeing, and research has found it to be related to better overall psychological health.[13] In addition, several models of psychotherapy teach clients strategies to strengthen an acceptance mindset, such as acceptance and commitment therapy (ACT) and dialectical behavioral therapy (DBT).

Confide in a Friend, Family Member, Clergy Member, Faith Healer, or Therapist

Amir's adult daughter has lived with depression, anxiety, and borderline personality disorder for many years. He struggles with guilt, wondering if he somehow caused her mental health problems or could have gotten her help earlier.

After his imam, his Muslim religious leader, spoke at the Friday call to prayer on mental health, Amir felt comfortable asking to meet with him. Amir found the meeting to be comforting, freeing, and empowering, as the imam helped him release his guilt and focus on supporting his daughter. Although Amir had found talking to his family to be helpful, the ability to share openly with an unbiased professional gave him new perspectives and a greater sense of peace.

Putting your feelings in words and sharing them with a trusted listener can help you understand your experience and feel less alone. Opening up can feel awkward and vulnerable, but your relationship with the other person may deepen as a result. It may be helpful to let the listener know how they can be most helpful, be it offering advice, just listening, or problem-solving together. You might also consider the benefits of connecting with a mental health professional who can offer objective, confidential support and guidance.

Practice Self-Compassion

Although Cheyenne isn't sure what mental illness her sister has, she knows it's very serious. Her sister has been living on the streets for several years. She reaches out for help only when she needs money or is in legal trouble. At those times, her sister talks in confusing ways, accuses Cheyenne of stealing, and appears to be responding to voices that no one else hears. Cheyenne worries a lot and is frustrated that her sister doesn't want professional help. Cheyenne has tried to start a civil commitment process in the past, but each time her sister has not met criteria.

Cheyenne read a book on self-compassion and found the messages to be comforting. She learned to (a) offer herself the same gentle kindness that she would give a friend who was hurting, (b) honor her own suffering, knowing everyone struggles at times, and (c) observe and accept her thoughts and feelings as they are—rather than ignoring them or blowing them out of proportion.[14] Being compassionate with herself was hard, and Cheyenne knew she would always advocate for her sister when she could. However, with the help of a good therapist and spiritual healer, she was able to be gentler with herself and more accepting of the situation.

Research on self-compassion has demonstrated that people who are kinder to themselves when facing emotional pain tend to have higher overall well-being and less emotional distress (depression, anxiety, stress).[14] Remembering that suffering is part of the human condition and relating to oneself with warmth rather than judgment can reduce the inner shame that often perpetuates painful emotions and drives social isolation. Dr. Kristin Neff is a well-respected leader in the area of self-compassion who has written numerous self-help books and has many helpful, free resources on her website (www.self-compassion.org).

How Are You Coping?

Now that you have read these stories, think about how you manage difficult situations and feelings. Perhaps you might be open to trying some new approaches.

If you find yourself turning to coping tools that are creating more problems such as gambling, excessive drinking, or illegal drug use, you may wish to connect with a peer support program, therapist, or primary care provider as well.

"Courage doesn't always roar: Sometimes courage is the little voice at the end of the day that says I'll try again tomorrow."

MARY ANNE RADMACHER[15]

Take a moment to write about your current coping tools and what you might try in the future. You might find some of the ideas in appendix B to be helpful. Be patient and have realistic expectations; even if a strategy helps by just 5%, that's progress.

Remember that self-care is not selfish—it's essential for your well-being. Scheduling time for yourself can make a big difference.

Your Coping Tools

What I do now:

- _____
  _____
- _____
  _____
- _____
  _____

What I will try in the next month:

- _____
  _____
- _____
  _____
- _____
  _____

Chapter 3

YOUR SUPPORT NETWORK

A LTHOUGH YOU KNOW THAT EVERYONE faces challenging, painful life situations, it's common to feel alone when supporting someone with a mental illness. Perhaps you worry that

I don't want to burden others with my problems. I don't want them to worry about me.

No one could understand what I'm going through unless they're also living it.

People would judge me if they knew how I really feel.

I don't want to burst into tears in front of my friends; they might feel uncomfortable and probably wouldn't know how to help anyway.

My problems aren't that bad compared to what other people face.

Denying your struggles (to yourself and others) and pretending that life is always rosy can lead to feeling even more isolated and lonely. A central message of this book is that you don't have to walk this journey alone.

IN THIS CHAPTER, YOU WILL

✓ Consider six facts about strong support networks

✓ Identify people you can count on

✓ Learn about potential benefits of support groups

✓ Reflect on sharing your journey with others

✓ Consider letting others know how they can support you

✓ Learn how an attorney may be a helpful member of your team

✓ Learn about the National Alliance on Mental Illness (NAMI)

Facts about Strong Support Networks

Let's start by considering these six facts:

FACT #1: Being socially isolated is just as bad for your health as smoking 15 cigarettes per day.[16]
Decades of research has found that having a strong support network is very important for both physical and mental health.[17] There are real health consequences of being socially isolated; the impacts are similar to how smoking cigarettes, drinking too much alcohol, and being physically inactive can affect our bodies, quality of life, and lifespan.[18] As the old song from the Broadway musical, *Funny Girl*, tells us: we are "People who need people."

FACT #2: Meaningful support is a lot different from the number of friends or followers you have on social media.
The meaning of "friend" has changed with social media. A meaningful friendship where you can be vulnerable and are seen, understood, valued, and accepted for who you are is totally different from the number of Facebook friends—or the number of "likes" an Instagram or TikTok post gets. One can have a thousand social media "friends" but still feel very lonely.

FACT #3: Reaching out and being honest with someone takes COURAGE.
Confiding in someone about your feelings and experience is a risk, and you may not always receive the support you are seeking. It's usually best to start slowly and see if the person is trustworthy before being too vulnerable. The level of detail that you share varies depending on the situation and relationship, but sometimes opening the door can lead to a meaningful interaction and friendship.

FACT #4: You may be surprised to learn that others can relate to your experience more than you would have imagined.

Because mental illness and trauma are so common, you might discover that the person you confide in can relate to your situation more than you anticipated. They may also love someone who has a mental illness or history of trauma and be grateful for your honesty. Your courage could allow them to share their experience as well; you might develop a connection where you both feel understood and supported.

FACT #5: There are many ways to reach out for support.

You can ask for support in many ways and from a wide variety of people. Although getting together in person has some advantages, issues such as physical distance, transportation, physical health, and busy schedules can make that difficult. Therefore, consider seeking support in other ways such as reputable blogs, social media groups, support groups (see below), and hotlines (see Resource List for specific numbers). You figure out what you want or need, and who can best support you at that time.

FACT #6: The truth is that not all of your friends or family members are able to provide meaningful support. Choose wisely and know who you can count on.

Some people are simply not able to be present, to understand, and to support you in your journey. This may be due to a variety of reasons, many having nothing to do with you or your loved one! The important task is for you to recognize when someone cannot provide meaningful support, find ways to interact with them that work for you (or consider taking a break from the relationship), and look elsewhere for validation and encouragement. Let's now turn to your current support network and think about how different people show up for you.

Who Can You Count On?

You likely turn to different people in your life for different reasons. For example, you may not call your 85-year-old grandma to go for a long hike in the woods, and you wouldn't invite your 10-year-old nephew out for happy hour. Instead of "putting all your eggs in one basket" and relying on a couple of people to meet all of your needs, it's good to have a variety of folks in your life. To avoid overwhelming your immediate family, it can be helpful to also reach out to folks who are less involved with your loved one and everyday life.

Who can you turn to when you want someone who

- Will just listen and not give unsolicited advice _____

- Can make you laugh _____

- Is comforting when you need to cry _____

- Gives good advice _____

- Has been though a similar situation so really understands _____

- Will help in a crisis any time, 24/7 _____

- Can handle your anger and not be overwhelmed _____

- Will pray or meditate with you . . . or just enjoy being quiet together _____

- Will send silly or supportive messages or memes during tough times _____

If you struggle to identify people who can show up for you, please be gentle with yourself. Making and maintaining friendships take work, and your energy may be depleted by supporting your loved one and family. If you are able to list one person who is a true friend, you are lucky indeed!

Also, remember the healing support and friendship you can get from pets. They can provide companionship, unconditional love, loyalty, and playfulness—all invaluable gifts.

Reaching Beyond Your Current Support Network: Support Groups

In addition to family and friends, you may find comfort and support in connecting with others who also understand your experience. Many wonderful organizations offer a range of courses and support groups regarding mental illness, and we encourage you to review them (appendix E). At the end of this chapter, we feature the National Alliance on Mental Illness (NAMI) due to its nationwide presence, provision of services and classes at no cost, and specific mission of supporting people living with all kinds of mental illness and their friends and family members.

If your loved one has problems with alcohol or drugs, you may also want to seek support in groups that specifically address those issues. Chapter 14 focuses on topics related to substance misuse, and the appendices describe several groups you and your loved one may find useful.

Sharing Your Journey with Others

In considering sharing your experience with others, you may wonder how your loved one would feel about it. This can be a tricky topic; there is no "one size fits all" approach. There is no rulebook on *if, what,* and *how* to share. It's possible that your needs may conflict with those of your loved one, and there's often no clear answer.

Understanding and Considering Your Loved One's Wishes

We encourage you to consider your loved one's wishes about what to share regarding their illness. A cornerstone principle of the recovery movement is a *person-centered approach.* This includes self-determination, in which the person with the mental illness defines their own goals and path; it also means having input into everything related to the illness and its treatment . . . including what is said and to whom.

So, we encourage you to talk with your loved one about their wishes. You may learn that they are:

OK WITH YOUR SHARING: Some people with mental health problems are comfortable openly discussing their illness and want family members and friends to do the same. Your loved one may recognize and worry about how their illness impacts you. They may want you to seek support for yourself.

NOT IN A GOOD PLACE TO HAVE THIS DISCUSSION: If your loved one is experiencing paranoia or anosognosia (they lack awareness of their illness—more on this in chapter 13), asking about sharing with others may wo7rsen their symptoms and increase the tension in your relationship. They may not understand why you would want support.

NOT OK WITH YOUR SHARING: Your loved one may not want others to know about their illness due to feelings of shame, embarrassment, desire for privacy, fear of judgment, and fear of discrimination. How do you as a family member or friend handle this situation? There are two schools of thought about this (see page 36).

Your loved one's feelings and preferences may change over time, so this can be an ongoing discussion. They may feel comfortable with your sharing with some people but not others. It can be helpful to seek to understand your loved one's concerns about disclosure and, at the same time, explain your need for support as well.

Regardless of your decision about sharing with family and friends, remember you can be assured of confidentiality when talking to a mental health professional (tips on finding

You don't talk about it

Pros

- Consistent with the philosophy of person-centered care, you respect your loved one's autonomy and wishes.

- Your loved one feels more in control and experiences you as trustworthy.

Cons

- You cannot receive help from your support network. They can't be there for you if they don't know what's going on.

- You may feel isolated and overwhelmed.

- It's harder to be involved in advocacy efforts.

- It takes a lot of energy to keep the secret.

You use discretion and share with a small number of trusted people . . . and ask them to respect your loved one's privacy

Pros

- You can draw upon your support network.

- You feel less alone.

- You have people to reach out to in a crisis (in addition to crisis resources as described in the Resource List).

- You can fight stigma around mental illness by talking openly about it.

Cons

- Your loved one may feel hurt and betrayed by your sharing without their permission (or against their wishes) . . .which can hurt your relationship.

one are offered in chapter 7). You can also get support from NAMI or other similar programs (see appendix F, Family Education Programs and Support Groups). Although maintaining confidentiality is a fundamental value in these groups, it cannot be guaranteed.

In summary, we acknowledge that this can be a delicate, sensitive issue. Your decision may be affected by your family and cultural norms, your relationship with your loved one, the nature of your loved one's illness, and their current level of functioning. We believe it's important to consider your loved one's wishes AND to be able to share your experience and get the support you need.

What To Share?

If you decide to share your experience with family members and friends, you may grapple with other questions such as: *What should I say? How much is too much? How will they react? Could they ever understand?*

What you say is totally up to you. You may decide to share your emotions—worry, exhaustion, frustration, sadness, powerlessness, hope. You may ask for support in dealing with tricky situations. Perhaps you simply want someone to listen. What you share definitely varies with each relationship and can change over time. At first, you may not know precisely how someone will respond, but you'll quickly get a good sense of their ability to show up: to be emotionally available, to try to understand your experience, and to support you and your family.

Letting Others Know
How They Can Support You

It can be helpful to let family members and friends know how they can be supportive. Although they likely want to show up for you, they may honestly not know how—and may fear upsetting you, crossing a boundary, or saying something offensive. Therefore, even if it feels a bit awkward, be *direct* and offer *specific* ways they can support you.

Of course, not everyone will respond to your requests; some people may distance due to their own issues or discomfort with the topic. Know that such withdrawal is probably not a reflection of you, but is most likely rooted in their own pain or history. Part of the benefit of support groups is the ability to connect with others who can truly understand your experience and are usually not overwhelmed by your challenges. So, if some of your existing friends are not able to be there for you, be open to new friendships.

Take a moment to reflect:

What have people done in the past that felt supportive for you? _____

_____

_____

When you're worried or upset about your loved one, how could others support you (perhaps providing a meal, taking the kids to the park, going on a walk together)? _____

_____

_____

Who might you ask for support this week—and how might they be able to help? _____

_____

_____

> "When my son was in the hospital for a psychotic break, I called two of his aunts and asked if they would visit him. They were happy to but didn't know what to do or what to say. I described what to expect when visiting a psychiatric unit and told them just to be themselves.
> That's all they needed to feel comfortable."
>
> —A DAD

Another Potential Member of Your Team: An Attorney

In addition to seeking support from your personal network and the health care system (more on that in chapter 7), you may benefit from obtaining legal advice. Depending on your loved one's level of functioning and financial situation, you might engage an attorney to explain your and your loved one's rights. They can help with petitioning for guardianship if appropriate; appointed guardians can make personal decisions for an individual who does not have capacity to maintain their own health and safety.

Some state laws allow the use of **psychiatric advance directives (PAD)**, which are legal documents that describe a person's preferences regarding future mental health treatment. The individual may designate someone (often termed a "proxy") to make treatment decisions on their behalf if they are in crisis and unable to do so. The National Resource Center on Psychiatric Advance Directives (www.nrc-pad.org) has up-to-date information by state on how to create these directives. You may also find the free mobile app, My Mental Health Crisis Plan, to be helpful in creating and sharing such a document.

Attorneys can also walk you and your loved one through the complicated process of applying for disability benefits. These details are beyond the scope of this book, but your loved one may be eligible for Supplemental Security Income (SSI) and Social Security Disability Insurance (SSDI). Although both programs pay benefits to people with disabilities, SSI is specifically for people with limited income and resources. SSDI funds are only available if the applicant (or a spouse or parent) has a qualifying work history, meaning having paid Social Security taxes on work earnings. You can learn more about applying for these benefits via phone (1-800-772-1213), the Social Security website (www.ssa.gov), or at your local Social Security office.

The National Alliance on Mental Illness (NAMI)

NAMI is a grassroots mental health organization with over 600 chapters located across the United States. Founded in 1979, it advocates for mental health and public policy and provides a wide range of free services for people with mental health concerns and those who love them.

Their vision statement is: "NAMI envisions a world where all people affected by mental illness live healthy, fulfilling lives supported by a community that cares."

Research has found that participating in the NAMI Family-to-Family Program helps people understand mental health issues, strengthens coping skills, and empowers participants to better advocate for their loved ones.[19]

Although each NAMI chapter is unique, common programs include

- **Educational Classes for Adults Who Care about Someone Living with Mental Health Concerns**
  - NAMI Family to Family: for those who care about an adult
  - NAMI Homefront: for those who care about a military service member or veteran
  - NAMI Basics: for parents or caregivers of youth with mental health concerns

- **Support Groups**
  - NAMI Family Support Group: for adults who love someone experiencing mental health concerns
  - NAMI Connection: for adults with mental health problems

- **Community Presentations and Events**
  - Presentations to raise awareness of mental illness and recovery
    » In Our Own Voice: for the general public
    » Ending the Silence: for middle and high school students
    » Sharing Hope: for African American communities
  - Annual NAMI Walk fundraisers
  - Annual conferences

- **Advocacy Opportunities and Training**
  - Advocacy campaigns such as #Act4Mental health and #Vote4MentalHealth that fight for affordable and effective treatment, early intervention, humane crisis response, parity for mental health care, combating stigma and discrimination, and more
  - Workshops teaching how to express your voice, share your story, and get involved in federal, state, and local advocacy efforts

NAMI also offers
- A helpline that offers free information and support about mental health services (phone: 800-950-NAMI; email: helpline@nami.org; text "helpline" to 62640)

- A book entitled *You Are Not Alone: The NAMI Guide to Navigating Mental Health*,[20] which describes NAMI programs and offers detailed information on mental health conditions and recovery. Psychiatrist Dr. Ken Duckworth draws not only from his decades of clinical work but also from his experience of having a father with bipolar disorder. Wisdom, guidance, and first-hand stories from experts and lay people are interspersed throughout the book.

"When I found NAMI, I felt like I was home—someone understood and cared.

There were no judgments or platitudes. I have many solid, long friendships, but I can't relax and feel heard with anyone like I can with my NAMI friends."

—A MOM

We encourage you to check out the NAMI website: www.nami.org. You can also follow a link to the NAMI state program nearest you to see what's available in your community.

Chapter 4

STIGMA AND DISCRIMINATION

I**T'S EASY TO SHARE GOOD NEWS** and pleasant emotions—excitement about a new job, happiness about a new romantic partner, or relief at remission of an illness. People in your support network usually respond positively in these situations, and they want to spend time together to hear more.

On the other hand, sharing struggles and emotional pain can be harder. People may not know what to say and may respond by distancing from you or being judgmental. Even if these responses don't happen, the fear that they might can be powerful. As a result, mental illness is sometimes kept silent or talked about in hushed tones.

Let's consider the following conversations you might have with your boss. Would your experience differ in each of these situations?

- *I need the afternoon off tomorrow to take my son to doctor appointment because he needs an adjustment on his medications for his*
  - *Chronic obstructive pulmonary disease*
  - *Bipolar disorder*

- *I need to take leave of absence to*
  - *Help my folks move into senior living facility due to Dad's memory problems*
  - *Care for my grandkids due to my daughter's mental health crisis*

- *I need to leave work immediately because I just got a text that my grandson*
  - *Was in a bad car accident*
  - *Took an overdose of his medications*

- *Let's get flowers for our co-worker who was just admitted to the hospital for a*
    - *A heart attack*
    - *A psychotic episode*

If these conversations would be different depending on the physical or mental health problem, the question is: Why is that so?

IN THIS CHAPTER, YOU WILL

Learn about stigma and discrimination surrounding mental illness, including

✓ Different types of stigma

✓ Causes of stigma and discrimination

✓ Potential consequences

✓ Strategies for coping

✓ Advocacy opportunities

Defining Stigma and Discrimination

Stigma is defined as negative **attitudes or beliefs** about people living with specific characteristics or engaging in certain behaviors. Many groups are stigmatized, such as people with a physical disability, mental illness, different body shape or size, and those who misuse substances. People who find themselves involved with the criminal justice system or those who struggle with poverty or unstable housing are also sometimes judged negatively.

Discrimination refers to **behaviors** that treat people unfairly due to their condition or situation. Discrimination sends a strong, judgmental message of exclusion—separating people from one another ("us" versus "them"). Discrimination can be obvious (such as bullying) or subtle (microaggressions such distancing from a friend who is having mental health problems). It can also be a lack of equitable access to health care, housing, and employment.

Stigma and Discrimination around Mental Illness

With respect to mental illness, stigma and discrimination can apply both to having the illness and to seeking professional help.

Stigma surrounding mental illness frequently reflects stereotypes or negative and inaccurate beliefs. Often grounded in fear and lack of understanding, the judgmental attitudes may relate to

- Ability or potential
  - *She could never hold down a job.*
  - *He'll always be like this—he can never get better.*

- Character
  - *He's just lazy and weak—he could do so much more if he wanted to.*
  - *She doesn't seem like the kind of person that would be depressed.*
  - *He may be dangerous.* (Fact: most people with a mental illness do not behave aggressively.)

- Mental health treatment
  - *They are weak for going go therapy—they should just get more friends.*
  - *He can just quit drinking anytime he wants to.*
  - *The antidepressant she's taking is addictive—it's just like cocaine.*

Remember that these messages are FALSE. Sadly, some people continue to hold these beliefs, and their words and behavior can be damaging.

Do you know if your loved one has encountered stigma—judgmental assumptions, reactions, or comments from others? If so, describe. _____

_____

_____

Are you aware if your loved one faced discrimination due to their mental illness? If so, describe. _____

_____

_____

What have you observed about how the stigmatizing or discriminating behaviors affected your loved one? _____

_____

_____

How did you feel when you became aware of these situations? _____

_____

_____

Types of Stigma

Although stigma is often seen as negative judgments from other people, it can also show up in other ways,[21] including

- Self-stigma

- Structural stigma

- Family or friend experience of stigma

Self-stigma (also known as "internalized stigma") refers to negative attitudes and shame about oneself due to having the illness. With this kind of stigma, people start to believe that the negative views they hear from others about mental illness apply to them. For example, some people doubt their abilities when they hear inaccurate stereotypes about mental illness. They may question why they should even try. These thoughts can damage confidence, self-esteem, ambition, and hope for the future.[22]

Do you sense that your loved one experiences shame or embarrassment about having a mental illness? _____

_____

_____

If so, what do you notice about how this self-stigma affects them? _____

_____

_____

Structural Stigma and Discrimination (also known as "institutional stigma") involves organizational or governmental policies, laws, and practices that limit opportunities for people with a mental illness. Examples of this kind of discrimination include less funding for mental health research than for other conditions, inadequate resources dedicated to mental health treatment; barriers to housing, and insurance company denial of covering mental health services due to being deemed not "medically necessary." The Paul Wellstone and Pete Domenici Mental Health Parity and Addiction Equity Act passed as federal law in 2008 and requires equal insurance benefits for mental health and substance misuse issues and other medical conditions. However, it does not apply to all health plans and is not uniformly followed. Structural stigma and discrimination often result in people not being able to afford, access, or continue with needed treatment.

Family or Friend Experience of Stigma (also known as "affiliated stigma") refers to people encountering stigmatizing attitudes and behavior because of their relationship with someone experiencing a mental illness.

For example, some family members and friends experience judgment (or fear others' judgment) for

- Causing the mental illness: *You must have been a bad parent.*

- Not doing enough (implying that you're responsible for their well-being): *You really should . . .*

- Being angry or impatient: *You should be more understanding—after all, they have a mental illness.*

- Being overly strict and setting limits: *Why won't you give them another chance?*

Have you ever felt judged or criticized due to your loved one's mental illness or substance misuse? If so, describe: _____

_____

_____

Have you been criticized for how you support your loved one? If so, what was that like for you? _____

_____

_____

Because of this stigma and the fear of others' judgment, some family members and friends feel ashamed and keep their loved one's illness private. Although keeping the secret is certainly a choice, as we discussed in chapter 3, doing so can take a lot of energy and can prevent you from receiving support from others.

Family members and friends can also experience stigma in rather subtle ways. For example, consider this situation faced by Janet and her family:

> When Janet's daughter was hospitalized due to leukemia, her friends and family really showed up. Meals were delivered, cards and flowers were sent, and a Caring Bridge site was set up to keep everyone up to date. Janet's brother created a GoFundMe page to help with medical expenses. Janet appreciated the outpouring of gifts and supportive messages.
>
> A few months later, Janet's husband, who has schizophrenia, started hearing voices quite intensely. His medicine wasn't working well. Seeing him so out of touch with reality was scary for Janet and their kids. He was in the hospital for several weeks but . . . no casseroles . . . no financial support. Very few offers to help. Everybody knew what was going on, but where were they? It hurt a lot.

The differences in how people respond to physical versus mental health crises can be striking and can reflect the stigma surrounding mental illness.

Have you experienced this more subtle type of stigma, such as people distancing from you or not being supportive during times of mental health crisis? If so, describe.

_____

_____

_____

Did it affect your relationships with those people? If so, how? _____

_____

_____

How did you deal with the situation? _____

_____

_____

Causes of Stigma and Discrimination

What do you think contributes to stigma surrounding mental illness? _____

_____

_____

People's attitudes and beliefs about mental illness are shaped by many factors, including but not limited to the following three factors.

Media: Sadly, the media often perpetuates negative attitudes and misinformation by portraying people with a mental illness as violent or dangerous. Words such as "crazy," "lunatic," and "retarded" send derogatory messages about people with mental health problems. Language that ridicules mental health professionals ("shrink") and treatments (e.g., "happy pills," "nut house," "straight jacket") also contributes to stigma.

Fear and lack of experience and education: As human beings, we often fear what we don't understand. We then avoid what is uncomfortable. When we keep a distance from people with a mental illness, we miss opportunities to form personal relationships that can enrich our lives and challenge negative stereotypes.

Some cultural norms and religious or spiritual belief systems: Some cultures view people with a mental illness as spiritual healers and shamans. In others, however, having a loved one with mental health concerns is a disgrace. Some believe that mental illness is caused by evil spirits and reflects weakness of character. Seeking psychotherapy is taboo and can bring shame to the family; people fear "losing face" with their elders. In addition, some cultures have generations of understandable distrust in the health care system due to past harmful treatment in the name of science or research. Therefore, stigma must be understood within each individual's unique cultural heritage and family system.

Consequences of Stigma and Discrimination

Stigma and discrimination themselves, as well as the **fear** of judgment and inequitable treatment, can have powerful consequences. Let's consider these emotions, thoughts, and behaviors experienced by some people who encounter stigma and discrimination related to their mental health (see figure below). Although this chart focuses on the person with the illness, family members and friends can have similar experiences. For

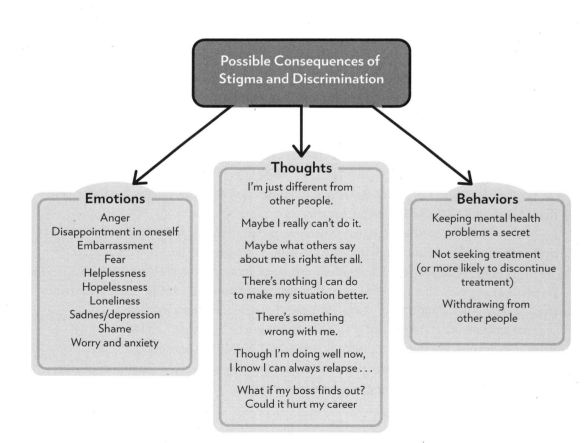

Possible Consequences of Stigma and Discrimination

Emotions
Anger
Disappointment in oneself
Embarrassment
Fear
Helplessness
Hopelessness
Loneliness
Sadnes/depression
Shame
Worry and anxiety

Thoughts
I'm just different from other people.

Maybe I really can't do it.

Maybe what others say about me is right after all.

There's nothing I can do to make my situation better.

There's something wrong with me.

Though I'm doing well now, I know I can always relapse . . .

What if my boss finds out? Could it hurt my career

Behaviors
Keeping mental health problems a secret

Not seeking treatment (or more likely to discontinue treatment)

Withdrawing from other people

example, encountering people who assume your loved one cannot do something because they have a mental illness may be painful. Watching your loved one suffer due to stigma and discrimination can be frustrating and heartbreaking.

Stigma and discrimination surrounding mental illness can lead people to suffer in silence and solitude. Although it takes courage to share openly with others, the experience of being seen, accepted, and supported can help challenge these emotions and self-limiting thoughts.

The truth is about one-third of American adults living with a serious mental illness do not receive professional mental health services.[23] Although many factors contribute to this stark reality, stigma and discrimination have long been recognized as major contributors. Sadly, without care, mental health problems can worsen and sometimes spiral to legal system involvement; substance misuse; and loss of housing, employment, and relationships.

Coping with Stigma and Discrimination

Although stigma and discrimination can be painful and have many negative outcomes, there are ways to manage and cope. In this section, we consider what you and your loved one can do in your own social networks, and the final part of this chapter describes broader advocacy opportunities.

- Surround yourself with people who will listen and refrain from judgment. If you encounter stigma or experience discrimination, seek support from someone who understands.

- Peer support groups can be especially helpful in combatting stigma and discrimination, both for mental illness and substance use problems. Groups offer opportunities to connect with others and challenge negative stereotypes. Check out appendices E and F for many helpful support programs.

- Remember that you and your loved one have choices surrounding disclosure of mental illness. See chapter 3 for an exploration of talking with others about your loved one's mental illness

- Be aware of the stigma surrounding mental health care and affirm your loved one for seeking help. (You may want to review chapters 6 and 7 where we offer tips on how to empower your loved one.)

- Remember that recovery is possible! Treatment can work, and more effective services are being developed every day.

- Remain hopeful. Recent large-scale national research has found some positive trends in public attitudes toward mental illness. For example, a recent survey studying changes in attitudes over time showed a significant decrease in the stigma surrounding depression.[24] Although stigma remains widespread and impactful, these improvements in public attitudes are encouraging.

Who has been most supportive of your loved one and their experience with mental illness? _____

_____

_____

How have they shown up? _____

_____

_____

Let's return to Janet and consider how she handled a tricky conversation with her friend, Carolyn:

> A few weeks after Janet's husband got home from the hospital, she contacted Carolyn, a friend who had been extremely supportive during her daughter's leukemia . . . but didn't reach out after her husband's hospitalization for a mental health crisis. Janet thanked Carolyn for all the meals and kindness during her daughter's illness. She also shared her hurt and disappointment when Carolyn didn't offer support with her husband's crisis. Carolyn listened and apologized; she said she had wanted to help but was uncomfortable—she didn't know what to do and feared saying or doing the wrong thing.
>
> Janet explained that families dealing with mental illness crises want a lot of the same support as when managing physical health emergencies . . . and that people distancing can add to the isolation and stigma around mental illness. Janet reassured Carolyn that it's OK that she doesn't understand schizophrenia or know exactly what to say. (She probably doesn't understand a lot about leukemia, either!) Janet shared that in the future she would appreciate Carolyn reaching out, listening, and just being there. Carolyn shared that she wants to overcome her discomfort with schizophrenia and she plans to do some reading about the illness. She appreciated Janet giving her feedback because she wants to be a supportive friend.

Advocacy

An additional, powerful way to challenge stigma and discrimination surrounding mental illness is through advocacy. Here are some of the ways you can advocate:

- **Consider sharing your story** when it feels appropriate.

- Express your perspectives related to mental health publicly via **social media, blogs, or letters to the editor.**

- Follow the legislature and **contact your state representatives** to share your experience and encourage them to support mental health bills.

- **Give feedback when you encounter stigmatizing messages,** either in the media or in everyday conversation.

- Use and encourage others to **use "people-first language."** Instead of referring to someone by their diagnosis (such as schizophrenic, borderline), use words such as: "has schizophrenia" or "living with borderline personality disorder."

- **Connect with local or national advocacy organizations,** like the National Alliance on Mental Illness (NAMI) as described in Chapter 3, to find ways to get involved.

Details surrounding advocacy organizations are provided in appendix D, Advocating to Fight Stigma and Discrimination.

> "Consider shining a light on *your* story—stigma festers in the dark and scatters in the light."
>
> **DEVIKA BHUSHAN, MD, FORMER ACTING SURGEON GENERAL OF CALIFORNIA**[25]

Chapter 5

NAMING LOSSES AND MOVING TOWARD ACCEPTANCE

B EING DIAGNOSED WITH ANY significant health condition—physical or mental—can be emotionally jarring. For some people and their families, getting a diagnosis can be a relief, as it may explain confusing symptoms and provide direction for helpful treatment. At the same time, people may experience a range of reactions that are commonly associated with grief and loss, such as when they

- Question, doubt, or deny the diagnosis

- Worry about the implications (*What does this mean for the future, relationships, job, finances, etc.?*)

- Resent the time, energy, and money associated with appointments, medications, and treatments

- Feel angry (*Why my loved one? Why me?*)

- Feel sad, depressed, or hopeless

These reactions can come and go over time as people hopefully move toward understanding and accepting the illness. When mental health problems are chronic and severe, the losses may be considerable. For example, despair may set in when people realize they may not attain their goals or fulfill lifelong dreams. Relationships and family life can be affected, which, when serious, may increase the risk of divorce or loss of custody of children. Financial, housing, and employment challenges may arise. Adult children may not be able to live independently and may return to the family home. Furthermore, as we discuss in chapter 4, these losses are often affected by the stigma and discrimination surrounding mental illness.

Has your loved one experienced losses associated with their illness? Roles they're no longer able to fulfill? Activities they're not able to do? If so, describe. And, what has that been like for you? _____

_____

_____

> "I'm angry that my daughter has this mental illness and addiction to cocaine. It's just not fair. Why her? She's lost so much . . . jobs, friendships . . . she even lost custody of her kids for a while. I know she's jealous of her friends who seem to have their lives "all together."
>   As for me, it just hurts to see her in such pain . . ."
>
> —A DAD

IN THIS CHAPTER, YOU WILL

✓ Reflect on your experience of loss, including potential loss or change in
  - Hopes for the future
  - Companionship in activities and family life
  - Feeling seen and supported
  - Emotional connection or intimacy

✓ Learn strategies to move toward acceptance

Your Experience of Loss

In addition to naming your loved one's losses, it's important to consider your experience as well. It may be tempting to downplay your feelings and minimize the many impacts on you, especially if you compare yourself to your loved one. Instead, we invite you to acknowledge and honor your process. If you notice yourself saying, "Well, at least I can . . . ," you may be discounting your feelings. Instead, please allow yourself to feel and accept whatever emotions arise as you reflect on your own losses.

A Note about Ambiguous Loss

Family therapist Dr. Pauline Boss, professor emeritus at the University of Minnesota, coined the term *"ambiguous loss."* [28] This involves grief surrounding your loved one being physically present but not emotionally available. They're "there" but "not there."

Although the term ambiguous loss was originally applied to dementia and traumatic brain injury, it applies to mental illness as well. Your loved one is just not the same person as before the illness. Accepting the many changes can be painful and you may miss the relationship you once had.

Four Kinds of Loss

Among people who love someone who experiences a mental illness, it's common to experience a sense of loss or change in the following four areas.

LOSS OR CHANGES IN HOPES FOR THE FUTURE

You may have long-standing dreams for your loved one, including goals for them individually and hopes for your relationship. Mental illness sometimes results in adjustments to these plans, which can be painful for everyone.

"I've always dreamed of my son graduating from college, getting married, and having kids. Because his symptoms of schizophrenia are so severe, I've had to let go of those hopes. The crushing sadness of seeing his former friends do all those things can be unbearable. I now focus on his strength and courage. I'm so proud of him."

—A MOM

Are there dreams you've had for your loved one that may not seem possible right now? If so, name them here if you like. _____

Any hopes for your relationship or future together that are no longer realistic? If so, name them here if you like. _____

For some families, another loss can pertain to finances. Depending on your specific situation, you may lose a partner's income or take on partial financial responsibility for your loved one. For example, your adult child may struggle financially: their disability payments aren't enough to live on, income from their part-time job doesn't cover their expenses, and the wait list for Section 8 housing is extremely long. In these situations, you may decide to help them financially and/or invite them to live with you, which may alter your own financial situation and future options. You might consider changing your career plan, working a greater number of hours or more years than planned, or holding down two jobs. You may have less money to put toward leisure activities or long-term goals. All of these changes can be part of your experience of loss and can be so very hard.

LOSS OF COMPANIONSHIP IN ACTIVITIES AND FAMILY LIFE

Over the years, perhaps you have shared everyday activities with your loved one, such as working out together at the gym, sharing in worship, going out to lunch, or cheering on the kids at soccer games. You may also have rituals such as annual family reunions and special holiday traditions. When your loved one's illness prevents them from participating in these activities, you may miss them and what they bring to these events. You might also just miss the companionship, as doing things by yourself can feel lonely.

> "It's so hard when my daughter can't come to our family holiday gatherings. Her anxiety is so crippling. She gets panicked when people ask questions about what she's doing with her life. I miss her so . . ."
>
> —A MOM

When your loved one does not attend a social event, you may face questions about where they are, which can be uncomfortable. You might not know how to respond. You might struggle with wanting to be honest while also respecting your loved one's privacy. To avoid these inevitable awkward questions, you might skip social events altogether. While staying home keeps you from having to face uncomfortable situations, you also miss opportunities to spend time with people you enjoy. So, either going solo or not going at all can be unsatisfying. One option is to take separate cars so your loved one can go home early if they wish. Other options are to go alone for a short period of time or confide in a friend who is attending for support. Yet another option is to be up front and directly say that your partner was not up to attending but you are glad you could make it. It's important for you to continue to engage socially even when your loved one is not able to participate.

How have you responded to questions about your loved one when they didn't attend a function or gathering? _____

_____

What was that like for you? _____

_____

What have you found helpful to say or do in those situations? _____

_____

> "My wife has never been able to attend our children's or grandchildren's sporting events due to her depression. Even though we have explained the depression to my daughter-in-law many times, she simply won't accept it or try to understand. It makes it much harder for me to deal with her on other things."
>
> —A HUSBAND

LOSS OF FEELING SEEN AND SUPPORTED

We often look to people we love to be present for us during both good and challenging times. It's normal and human to want our loved ones to

- Lift us up and offer compliments: *I'm proud of you for getting a black belt in karate; I know you've been working really hard.*

- Express care and love: *I'm so lucky to have you as my best friend.*

- Celebrate with us: *It's great you got a promotion at work; let's go out to celebrate!*

- Be dependable and trustworthy: *I know I can count on you as a brother and good friend to keep private what I share.*

- Provide support when we're struggling: *I'm so sorry that your sister died—I know how close you were.*

To what extent is your loved one able to "show up" emotionally for you right now?

How do you feel when they're unable to do so?

How do you cope with those situations?

Who can you turn to when your loved one is not able to support you? You may want to review the people that you identified in chapter 3.

When your loved one is experiencing an especially difficult time, they may seem quite self-focused. It's possible they aren't able to consider how their experience and actions affect you; they may not be able to offer you emotional support. Your relationship can feel one-sided during such times, leaving you feeling confused, hurt, and angry . . . and maybe sometimes invisible. Your loved one's emotional unavailability can be a painful loss.

You're not being selfish in wanting their comfort, love, attention, and support.

Let's meet Marilyn as she encounters unexpected issues with her partner, Dave:

Dave and Marilyn met in a grief support group shortly after their spouses died. They dated for a year and then honored their relationship with a commitment ceremony. Things were going well until Dave had a car accident and developed severe back problems, resulting in him being a wheelchair-user. He became very depressed as he mourned the loss of his spouse, his independence, and the ability to fish and hunt. He worried about the cost of his medications and often said he had no reason to get out of bed.

Watching Dave basically stop living is very hard for Marilyn. When they first met, he doted on her, they had long talks, and they supported each other with life's ups and downs. Now, she spends her days trying to lift his spirits and helping him manage his doctor appointments, medications, and insurance statements. He is no longer tender or attentive to her feelings, and she often feels like his nurse rather than his partner. This is not what she signed up for! She is afraid of being pulled down emotionally but stays active with her bridge club and precious grandchildren.

LOSS OR CHANGE IN EMOTIONAL CONNECTION OR INTIMACY

Mental illness can affect not only your experience of feeling seen by your loved one but how you connect emotionally and physically as well. Some people living with a mental illness avoid eye contact, speak in a flat manner without much emotion, and have little energy. It can be hard to feel close to someone who communicates in this way. It may feel like your loved one is there, but not there . . . part of the experience of ambiguous loss.

This emotional flattening can be part of the mental illness (especially depression and schizophrenia), a reaction to trauma (perhaps part of PTSD), or a side effect of a mental health medication. On the other hand, some people with bipolar disorder and some personality disorders experience and express emotions very strongly, which can be overwhelming for those around them. In either case, you may feel shut out, confused, hurt, or sad.

"Ever since my older brother got home from Iraq, he's had a thousand-yard stare. He drifts in and out of our conversations. I have no idea what he's thinking, but I know he's haunted by bad memories. He seems so far away emotionally, and I miss the friend who went away to war."

—A BROTHER

In intimate relationships, the changes in physical and sexual intimacy can also be a loss. Your loved one may have less (or more) interest in sexual activity. Furthermore, some mental health medications have side effects that can affect interest in sexual activity and sexual functioning. We offer some tips in chapter 11 on how couples can work together in enjoying emotional and physical intimacy.

Recognizing that your relationship has changed over time, are there activities you and your loved one do together that help you feel connected? If so, what?

_____

_____

_____

Do you miss ways in which you used to connect? If so, describe what you miss.

_____

_____

_____

Might there be other ways that you and your loved one could strengthen the emotional connection in your relationship? If so, how? _____

_____

_____

Chapter 8, Strengthening Your Connection, provides many tools for improving your bond with your loved one. If this kind of loss resonates with you, be sure to check out that chapter.

In addition to these four kinds of losses, have you experienced other losses in this journey with your loved one? If so, describe them. _____

_____

_____

Reflecting on These Losses

Reading about these painful losses may have been difficult. Take comfort in knowing that these feelings are real, understandable, and shared by many people. In other words, you are not alone.

Naming losses can give you power. It's no longer a vague, fuzzy feeling in your stomach or a dark cloud overhead; you can specifically describe the loss. Putting words to your experience can help navigate your emotions and make decisions about how to cope with them, including the possibility of acceptance.

Also, depending on your loved one's specific situation, remember that the losses may be temporary . . . or they may not always be quite as limiting as they are right now. During times your loved one is doing well, you can hopefully enjoy quality time together and reconnect emotionally.

Reminder: As you grieve these losses, be sure to draw upon connections with other people in your life. You can seek validation, friendship, and encouragement in many different relationships (in addition to your loved one—not instead of). Consider joining group activities, such as a community choir, bowling league, volunteering, or book club. Surround yourself with people who affirm and celebrate you (remember the people you identified in chapter 3). You can give and receive love in many ways—children, grandchildren, siblings, parents, pets, friends . . . be open!

Moving toward Acceptance

In this chapter we have reviewed several losses you might experience in your journey, which can involve emotional losses, financial changes, and perhaps unanticipated yet considerable commitments of your time and energy. You may feel sad and dearly wish your loved one did not have the illness. Perhaps you ask yourself, "Why me?" and question why you and your loved one must deal with this hard situation. At times you feel overwhelmed—all perfectly understandable feelings.

Now we invite you to consider what it means for you to accept the current reality of your loved one's mental illness. This is the coping tool that Enrique from chapter 2 was practicing with his son who was managing anxiety and drug misuse.

Acceptance involves acknowledging and honoring difficult situations and feelings and giving up the fight to try to change things beyond your control. With acceptance often comes adjusting expectations and goals and meeting your loved one where they are right now. Two reminders that can aid you in developing an intentional mindset of acceptance are

- The course of the illness may be hard to predict. Instead of waiting for some hoped-for tomorrow, you can help your loved one by being present with them in the here and now—and being available and supportive over time.

- Mental illnesses are complex conditions, and scientists are still learning about causes and effective treatments. Just as we would not ridicule someone with asthma by telling them to "just breathe better," urging someone living with depression to "just try harder" is neither helpful nor respectful.

Acceptance is rarely a one-time event and may take repeated intentional decisions. It is also not an all-or-nothing process, as some aspects of the situation may be easier to accept than others. Importantly, acceptance of situations you cannot change does not mean giving up hope or discontinuing being an advocate—not at all! On the contrary, accepting the reality can allow you to move forward and have more energy to support your loved one.

Consider these tips in helping to move toward acceptance:

A: Acknowledge the reality of the loss(es) associated with your loved one's illness
C: Concentrate on what you DO have control over
C: Choose gratitude
E: Empower and encourage your loved one
P: Provide yourself with the same comfort and compassion you'd offer a friend
T: Take one day at a time

A: Acknowledge the reality of the loss(es) associated with your loved one's illness. Name the losses that you, your loved one, and your family have experienced. Avoid judging the losses, but simply identify them and reflect on how they have impacted you.

C: Concentrate on what you DO have control over. It's likely that you have strong feelings about what's beyond your control. It's easy to get stuck in anger, helplessness, catastrophic thinking, and a downward spiral of unanswerable questions. However, after acknowledging your feelings, you can choose to focus on what you do have control over and put your energy there. You may try to calm your spirit with relaxation tools, physical exercise, journaling, therapy, or connecting with friends/family. You may also give yourself positive messages such as

- *I can manage hard situations.*
- *I can stay focused on the present instead of dwelling on the past or worrying about the future.*
- *I will get through this.*

C: Choose gratitude. Decades of research demonstrate the power of gratitude for well-being and relationships.[26] What are you grateful for? As you strive for acceptance, you might choose to intentionally focus on

- Your loved one's strengths and abilities
- The enjoyable parts of your relationship
- Good days (or weeks, months, or years)
- Progress, even if it's slow and not linear
- Your support network (personal and health care team)

E: Empower and encourage your loved one. Just as focusing on strengths, hope, and gratitude can be helpful for your own reflection, they're also great topics to discuss openly with your loved one. Honoring their efforts, abilities, courage, and progress can be powerful, both for their well-being and for your relationship. Your genuine compliments may mean more to them than you could imagine. Chapters 6 and 8 offer many ideas about how to be encouraging.

> ## "Talk to yourself as you would someone you love."
>
> **BRENE BROWN**[27]

P: Provide yourself with the same comfort you'd offer a friend. Realizing that accepting the situation can be painful, it's important to be kind to yourself. We describe strategies you might find helpful in chapter 2 and appendix B (Activities to Lift Your Spirit), including the idea of extending yourself the same compassion you would give a loved one or friend. You might consider what you would say to a friend who is in your situation . . . and then intentionally give yourself those same kind messages.

T: Take one day at a time, and never give up hope. Your journey of coping with losses and working toward acceptance can feel overwhelming at times. It is usually not linear. Take one day at a time. If a full day is too much, consider one hour or minute at a time.

Writing Opportunity

Writing can be a helpful tool for working through losses and moving toward acceptance. Consider writing your loved one a letter. Importantly, this is NOT to be shared with them. We want you to feel comfortable expressing your thoughts and feelings without censoring or worrying about your loved one's reaction.

Use this space if you wish, or use a personal journal or digital device if you prefer. These phrases may be helpful in getting started.

To focus on your feelings about the losses

I miss spending time with you doing . . .

I'm sad that . . .

I want you to know that . . .

Sometimes I feel distant from you which is . . .

I hope that . . .

To emphasize your support and acceptance of your loved one

Even though this is hard, we will get through this together because . . .

You are so much more than your illness, and I really admire . . .

I love spending time with you doing . . .

I love how you . . .

I'm so grateful . . .

I am so proud of you for . . .

I know you're doing the best you can . . . I see you . . . I believe in you . . . I . . .

Part II

SUPPORTING YOUR LOVED ONE

Chapter 6

EMPOWERING YOUR LOVED ONE IN LIVING THEIR BEST LIFE

*Working toward Goals and
Connecting with Other People*

T o EMPOWER SOMEONE IS TO support them in living their best life and moving toward their goals.

EMPOWERMENT IS NOT

- doing something "for" or "to" your loved one

- telling them what they "should" or "should not" do

- trying to "fix" or "change" them

EMPOWERMENT IS

- loyally walking alongside

- offering encouragement

- avoiding judgment

- celebrating progress

- being patient

- maintaining hope

- listening

- accepting where they are and simultaneously remembering their potential

Emotional health and well-being are more than simply the absence of symptoms. As a family member or close friend, you want to empower your loved one in their overall wellness. We encourage you to listen for and support *their* goals, wishes, and dreams . . . what they find important and meaningful.

Sometimes it's hard to know how to be supportive. You may struggle with questions such as

- *How can I offer support without nagging?*

- *How can I figure out what is doing "too much" versus being supportive and helpful?*

- *What should I encourage my loved one to do for themselves?*

- *How can I be their family member/friend but not their therapist?*

- *How can I encourage my loved one to consider new ideas or activities without taking responsibility for the outcome?*

- *What can I do when they don't want my input and help?*

> "I struggle figuring out how much to do for my son—I don't want to do TOO much—but I need to make sure he gets to work, fills out all his papers for the government on time so he doesn't lose his benefits, etc."
>
> —A MOM

Ultimately, it's helpful to encourage your loved one to do as much as possible for themselves. You also want to avoid becoming enmeshed in your loved one's life and potentially overwhelmed yourself (more on limit setting in chapter 10). Although stepping back can be hard, you're absolutely still available as a safety net and supporter. In the long-run, promoting their independence and self-reliance is important.

All of this can be a juggling act, and what is helpful can change across time and situation. During a crisis, you may be very involved and help navigate routines such as parenting, work, or household responsibilities (more on managing crises in chapter 16). However, other times you may be much less engaged, such as when they're doing well, when they don't desire your support, or when you set limits for yourself. So, it's helpful to be flexible and responsive to their current needs as well as your own.

IN THIS CHAPTER, YOU WILL

✓ Consider uplifting messages you might share with your loved one (as well as potentially hurtful ones to avoid)

✓ Gain tools for how to empower your loved one in their recovery as they
  ○ Set and work toward goals
  ○ Build relationships and engage with the community

✓ Reflect on times when your loved one didn't want your input and ways to manage those situations

Empowering versus Potentially Hurtful Messages

When thinking about communicating with your loved one, remember that words are powerful. They can encourage and reassure and, just as quickly, can humiliate and tear someone down.

Empowering Messages

The messages on the next page can help your loved one feel heard, empowered, and understood. Sharing these sentiments can also strengthen your relationship.

Remember: Although words can be powerful, sometimes just being present and listening can be the most helpful thing you can do. Spending time together in a relaxed manner can be comforting. You may consider things that don't require a lot of interaction or conversation, such as watching a sporting event or going for a drive. Chapter 8 offers many ideas of possible activities you may enjoy doing with your loved one.

WHEN YOU WANT TO	CONSIDER THESE MESSAGES
Instill hope	I believe in you. You've gotten through hard times in the past. You can do this.
Express empathy	That must be really tough. I know you're hurting. I'm sorry you're going through such a difficult time.
Remind them of their purpose and importance	You make such a difference in our family. You mean so much to me. You are so good at _____ You have such a caring heart. You matter!
Express your love, patience, and unwavering support	I'm here for you; we're in this together. I promise I won't judge you or your choices. I have not been in your shoes but want to try to understand. There's no rush. Take your time. I see you. I love you.
Ask how you can be supportive	I want to show up for you but am not sure how to do so. How can I support you? I'm on your team. Please let me know if there are any ways I can be there for you.
Respect a boundary	I understand if you want some space right now. If you don't want to talk, I understand. I'm here if you change your mind.
Remind them they're not alone	You're never alone—I'm here for you. You have so many people who care about you.
Offer physical affection	Could I give you a hug? How about a high five?

Potentially Hurtful Messages to Avoid

Some people don't understand mental illness and don't know what to say to someone who is struggling. You probably have heard uninformed, dismissive, and critical remarks. Although such comments may be intended to be helpful, they can be experienced as judgmental and insensitive; your loved one may feel misunderstood, sad, hurt, angry, or alone. Consider these messages:

Just get over it.

It's all in your head.

I know how you feel.

Quit feeling sorry for yourself.

It could be worse.

No one gets a free ride.

When are you going to move on? Just forget about it!

It's not that bad—pick yourself up and get going.

We've all been there.

Stop over-reacting and being so dramatic.

You look fine to me. Stop complaining.

You should appreciate your blessings—you have so much to be grateful for.

You have no reason to be depressed.

Get a hobby.

You just need to try harder.

Look on the bright side.

But you don't seem depressed.

*You're **still** seeing a therapist?*

Everything happens for a reason.

You're not the only one with problems.

Others you have heard: _____

If you ever feel tempted to make remarks such as these, get some distance and return when you are able to speak in a calm and respectful manner.

These messages can be hurtful because your loved one may already struggle with similar doubts and worries. Your loved one may desperately want to "get over it" and may be frustrated because they also think they "have no reason to be depressed." Hearing these comments from others can make people question themselves and feel even worse.

Having explored the importance of expressing affirming messages, the rest of this chapter offers specific tips for empowering your loved one with setting goals and engaging with the community.

Empowering Your Loved One in Their Recovery

Historically, the term "recovery" focused on discontinuing misuse of alcohol and drugs; however, the concept's meaning has broadened considerably. The Substance Abuse and Mental Health Services Administration (SAMHSA) now defines "recovery" from mental health and substance use problems as: "A process of change through which individuals improve their health and wellness, live a self-directed life, and strive to reach their full potential."[29] They name four major dimensions that support recovery, including

- **Health:** Overcoming or managing symptoms and making healthy choices that support well-being

- **Home:** Safe place to live

- **Purpose:** Meaningful daily activities

- **Community:** Supportive relationships

"Recovery is not a destination . . . (it) is living a full and meaningful life"

KATHERINE PONTE, JD, MBA, MENTAL HEALTH ADVOCATE AND CERTIFIED PSYCHIATRIC REHABILITATION PRACTITIONER[30]

In the past, treatment for mental illness largely focused on health—namely, symptom management. However, recovery means much more than just that; the strengths-based, culturally sensitive, hopeful, and trauma-informed concept of recovery today reflects the importance of many other aspects of well-being, including housing, purpose, and community.

A variety of specific recovery approaches have been developed, such as Dr. Mary Ellen Copeland's Wellness Recovery Action Plan (WRAP: www.wellnessrecoveryactionplan. com) and the Illness Management and Recovery (IMR) program.[31] These models guide people in creating structured, personalized plans that may include general wellness tools, daily maintenance practices, identification of stressors, use of social support, awareness of warning signs, and crisis and post-crisis planning. Themes of advocacy, hope, education, support, responsibility, and goal-setting are foundational elements of these approaches.

The rest of this chapter focuses on two of these key dimensions, including

- **Purpose:** Setting and working toward goals
- **Community:** Building relationships and engaging with the community

The next chapter offers guidance on how to empower your loved one in the health care system.

A brief yet important caveat: The potential success of all of these tips about strengthening your loved one's sense of purpose and community is contingent on their desire for your involvement. Although you can be an incredibly loving and supportive friend or family member, these actions are ultimately their decision. Taking on excessive responsibility as a caregiver and pushing them to follow these suggestions may result in considerable push-back from your loved one and burnout for you. Definitely tricky tensions to navigate . . . more on this at the end of the chapter.

Let's look at the Robinson family. We will follow their story throughout this chapter.

Alexis and Jasmine Robinson are sisters and have always been close. Alexis makes jewelry and has wanted to start her own business for several years. Now that she finished her associate degree, she's ready to begin. She wants to sell her jewelry online and at art shows. However, she has significant depression as well as frequent panic attacks; she lives in a chronic state of worry, wondering when another attack might happen. In addition, she has no idea how to start a business so turns to Jasmine for help.

Setting and Working toward Goals

If your loved one wishes your help, three ways to empower them in strengthening their sense of purpose include

- Support them in setting and making progress on goals

- Offer to help create a schedule with meaningful activities

- Instill hope and honor their strengths

Support in Setting and Making Progress on Goals

When opportunities arise and your loved one seems open to talking, ask about their hopes for the future—talk about what's important to them. When they share, listen for their values and what gives their life meaning. Having such ongoing discussions can give you insight into how to support them.

You can empower your loved one with their goals in many ways:

- Help to clearly define the goal, being as specific as possible
  - Remember that setting big, vague, and unattainable goals can result in feeling discouraged and unmotivated.
  - At the same time, goals should be challenging enough to engage and motivate your loved one.
  - Your role is to help your loved one consider options and make choices—not to decide for them.

- Think through and possibly write out the long-term goal and vision

- Define small, specific action steps they can start today
  - Progress on smaller steps can boost confidence and momentum to keep moving forward.

- Celebrate *effort, courage,* and *progress* rather than outcomes with phrases such as
  - *It took a lot of courage for you to . . .*
  - *I'm really proud of you for . . .*
  - *I know you put a lot of hard work into . . .*

- Remind them of their strengths (more on that in the next section)

- Brainstorm together how to overcome obstacles when they arise

Consider how Jasmine helps her sister with her goal of launching a jewelry business.

Alexis feels panicky and overwhelmed when she thinks about all the work involved in creating a business. Jasmine suggests they work together to define her goals and vision.

My Long-Term Goals and Vision: Create and launch my jewelry business, Art by Alexis

- Triple my collection of jewelry designs

- Sell my goods at art shows

- Hire a web designer to create a website to sell my product

- Develop a social media campaign to advertise my jewelry

Next, they talk through the details of Alexis' plan, create a timeline, and identify action steps. They decide to start small for the first year and then launch a website with online sales the following year.

My First-Year Goals

- Design and produce 10 new earring–necklace sets

- Have coffee with Uncle Darryl, an accountant, to get advice on creating a business plan

- Have a booth at three local art shows this summer

The sisters periodically review the plan, track progress, and troubleshoot challenges. They define their next steps and celebrate the progress to date.

Offer to Help Create a Schedule with Meaningful Activities

When working toward goals, having a predictable schedule can be helpful. Some people procrastinate or struggle emotionally when they don't have much structure. Having too much time with nothing to do can worsen depression, anxiety, and loneliness. A set routine can also facilitate personal accountability and progress.

If your loved one is open to your help, you might consider the following tips:

- Create a weekly schedule together (important for your loved one to lead this process)

- Start by adding existing routines such as regular sleep, exercise, relaxation time, therapy

- Build in fun, meaningful activities that you can enjoy together or that they can do with friends or other family members

- Be careful that the schedule doesn't get too busy

Brief Note about Sleep

Sleep is strongly connected to emotional health, and many people managing a mental illness struggle with getting quality, consistent rest. Although beyond the scope of this book, there are strategies that can help with sleep such as regular bedtime and wake time; avoiding naps; calming evening routines; avoiding screen time before bed; and having a dark, quiet, and cool bedroom. In addition, there is a highly effective treatment called Cognitive Behavioral Therapy for Insomnia (CBT-I). If your loved one struggles with sleep, encourage them to talk with their providers about possible treatment options.

Brief Note about Physical Activity

Just like sleep, the importance of regular physical activity cannot be overstated. Although expert guidelines suggest about 20 minutes a day of moderate-intensity aerobic activity,[40] doing any amount of physical activity is better than none. Physical activity has been shown to be highly effective in improving mental health[41] and can be a powerful part of an overall treatment plan and well-being. Your loved one may want to check with their family doctor before starting any significant exercise plan, and it is wise to start small with light activities such as short walks. It's important for your loved one to find something they enjoy, so perhaps offer to try out different activities together.

- Be flexible and adapt (Sometimes life happens and schedules need to change—that's OK! This schedule is intended to be a general guide, not rigid or stressful.)

- Post the schedule somewhere visible, such as on the fridge

- Review the schedule each week and add upcoming events

Instill Hope and Honor Their Strengths

Creating new routines and working toward goals take courage. It's easy to lose motivation when challenges arise. As a family member or friend, you can empower your loved one by being hopeful. Remember the phrases listed in the beginning of this chapter that convey your belief in them.

You may also honor and remind your loved one of their strengths. Many people with a mental illness share how their experiences have enabled them to further develop their strengths, such as courage, vulnerability, and empathy for others.[32]

Consider the following list of qualities and circle those that describe your loved one (some items adapted from VIA Character Strengths).[33]

Appreciates beauty	Generous	Loyal
Brave	Good sense of humor	Open-minded
Caring about others	Grateful	Passionate
Creative	Honest	Perceptive
Compassionate	Hopeful	Resilient
Curious	Humble	Sensitive
Dedicated	Kind	Spiritual
Fair	Loves to learn	Tender
Forgiving	Loving	Thoughtful

What other strengths do you admire in your loved one? _____

_____

_____

How often do you tell them that you notice and appreciate these qualities? _____

_____

_____

How do they respond when you genuinely affirm their strengths? _____

_____

_____

"I believe that our struggles can be the source of our superpowers. They show us our capacity for vulnerability and strength—that we can endure and overcome hard things. They also give us empathy for the full spectrum of human experience, allowing us to better support others at their most vulnerable moments."

DEVIKA BHUSHAN, MD, FORMER ACTING SURGEON GENERAL OF CALIFORNIA[32]

Note: As we discuss in chapter 8, focusing on your loved one's strengths can also help your relationship. Human beings tend to *find* what we look for. When frustrated, it's easy to focus on irritating behaviors. However, being intentional about celebrating good qualities and progress on goals can not only boost their self-esteem, but can bring you closer, such as with the Robinson sisters.

> Jasmine knows that starting a business is a big undertaking. She reminds Alexis of her artistic gifts and shares how proud she is. When Alexis faces setbacks, Jasmine encourages her, focusing on her creativity and effort. Jasmine knows that Alexis derives a lot of satisfaction from her art and wants to help her in any way she can.
>
> There have been times, however, when Alexis has resented Jasmine's offers and wanted to do things on her own. When that happened, Jasmine gave her space but felt confused and worried. She simply didn't know what to do, so just waited for Alexis to reach out again.

Building Relationships and Engaging with the Community

If your loved one is open to your support in building relationships and connecting with the community, you might consider the following strategies:

- Enjoy rituals together

- Encourage community involvement

- Suggest connecting with peers

Enjoy Rituals Together

Rituals are meaningful activities you do regularly, often with people you care about. They can be everyday routines such as eating dinner as a family or resting together on Saturdays in honor of the Sabbath. Rituals can be creative such as Taco Tuesdays or Sunday Movie and Popcorn Night. Friends, too, can enjoy rituals such as nature walks together on Sunday afternoons. Regardless of the activity, rituals can be fun, something predictable to look forward to, a way to strengthen relationships, and a source of lasting memories.

What rituals do you have with your loved one? _____

If you don't have many rituals now, what might your loved one enjoy? (Perhaps you could brainstorm some ideas together.) _____

Encourage Community Involvement

In 2023, Dr. Vivek Murthy, the United States Surgeon General, termed the "loneliness epidemic" a public health crisis, and created a national action plan to promote social connection.[34] Even before the COVID pandemic, about half of all US adults reported considerable loneliness. Further, people living with a serious mental illness experience higher rates of loneliness than the general population.[35] Research has documented many health consequences of feeling lonely and being socially isolated, such as an increased risk of heart disease, stroke, depression, anxiety, and premature death.[36]

Because mental illness can feel very isolating, encouraging social connections can be important. Dr. Thomas Insel, psychiatrist and former director of the National Institute of Mental Health, says that recovery from a mental illness involves the "3Ps," namely *people, purpose, and place* (housing).[37] Participation in work, volunteering, and other meaningful activities can contribute to this sense of *purpose* and can build connections with other *people*.

Is your loved one engaging with others in the community now; if so, how? _____

_____

_____

Do you notice it making a difference in their well-being? If so, how? _____

_____

As you talk with your loved one about getting involved in the community, listen for their concerns. Ask specifically about potential barriers, such as anxiety and bad past experiences. Consider how their symptoms (such as low energy, social anxiety, low self-confidence, delusional beliefs) may be obstacles. Finding something they are willing to try can take a long time, so be patient and keep planting seeds.

While acknowledging their concerns, you may discuss a wide range of possible benefits of community involvement, such as opportunities to

- Make friends

- Have fun

- Use their skills

- Remember their meaning and purpose in life

- Have more routine and structure

- Distract from their own concerns

- Help somebody else

How your loved one might engage with the community depends on their interests, preferences, and well-being. Some general options are listed below, and mental health providers can suggest local resources. Although in-person activities have advantages, some people may find remote or virtual participation more comfortable, especially at the beginning.

- Volunteering
  - Many national and local websites have lists of current opportunities, such as www.volunteermatch.org.
  - Mental health organizations such as the National Alliance for Mental Illness (NAMI) offer low-stress, flexible roles for volunteers.

- Work
  - It's helpful to explore flexible, low-stress work activities and possibly start with a few hours per week.
  - Supported Employment, such as Individual Placement and Support (IPS), is an excellent research-based model for helping people with a mental illness succeed in mainstream, competitive jobs.[38] See appendix E for more information. Your loved one could ask their mental health provider about available services in their community.

- Exercising at a gym or fitness center with others
  - As noted earlier, physical activity is excellent for both physical and emotional well-being.
  - Having a work-out buddy, personal trainer, or scheduled fitness class can help with motivation and accountability and can offer opportunities for friendship.
  - As some mental health medications have side effects that affect physical health (such as weight gain and drowsiness), regular exercise can be especially useful for overall well-being.

- Community education classes or groups
  - Classes can provide opportunities to learn skills, meet new people, and just have fun.
  - Many community building websites allow you to search a topic to find other people with similar interests (such as MeetUp.com). These groups often offer both online and in-person events, and connecting with people who care about the same things you do can be enjoyable.

- Church/house of worship activities
  - If your loved one finds meaning or enjoyment in spiritual or religious activities, participation in a church or house of worship can build community,
  - As large events may be overwhelming, small classes or activities may feel more comfortable,

Let's check in on Alexis and Jasmine.

> The sisters have a ritual of meeting at the coffee shop every Sunday afternoon. It's time for them to reconnect and review progress.
>
> The sisters find a Meetup specifically for female small business owners. Alexis is relieved to see that the group offers virtual meetings, because going in person feels daunting and nerve-racking. Alexis looks forward to networking with other women who have started their own companies. They agree that Jasmine will text Alexis shortly before the first meeting to offer encouragement.
>
> After attending her first meeting, Alexis called Jasmine to share her excitement. She had fun and got some great ideas from people who had sold products at art shows and online. The other women raved about the hand-made earrings Alexis wore that night—they asked to see pictures of her other jewelry. Alexis was pleased that her anxiety was pretty manageable during the meeting, and she thought about going to next month's meeting in person.

Suggest Connecting with Peers

When managing a mental illness, connecting with others who "get" your experience can help decrease isolation and foster hope. Your loved one may enjoy meeting people who understand their journey, such as peer support specialists and members of support groups. Clubhouses can also provide rich opportunities for building relationships.

Peer support specialists are people with lived experience of mental illness who receive formal training in helping others. Specialists draw upon and share their own recovery experience as they help people learn skills, manage crises, access health care, advocate for services, and develop recovery plans. They sometimes work individually with people in hospitals, clinics, and prisons, and jails; in addition, they are integrated into team-based care models such as crisis response teams. Peer specialists can be empowering role models and friends for those in the throes of difficult times. Promising research is documenting how peer support interventions are associated with reductions in mental health symptoms and improvements in overall personal recovery, such as a sense of purpose, empowerment, and hope.[39]

Peer support groups offer opportunities to give and receive support from others who manage similar challenges. Group members can offer encouragement, hope, nonjudgmental listening, resources, and friendship. Many support groups are available, including programs specifically focused on mental illness (e.g., National Alliance on Mental Illness, NAMI; Depression and Bipolar Support Alliance, DBSA) and substance misuse (e.g., 12-step programs like Alcoholics Anonymous). Appendix E (Mental Health Treatments and Services for Your Loved One) includes details and contact information for many peer support programs.

Clubhouses are community centers that provide many supports and services for people with a mental illness. Individualized plans are developed, and members are supported with their recovery goals such as finding housing, landing a job, or getting additional training. Grounded in a spirit of peer support, hope, mutual respect, and empowerment, clubhouses can provide a sense of belonging, meaningful relationships, social activities, and access to crisis services when needed. To find a clubhouse in your area, see the Clubhouse International website: www.clubhouse-intl.org

When Your Loved One Doesn't Want Your Input

Empowering your loved one isn't always easy, especially when they are not interested in your suggestions. You may feel discouraged when your recommendations are dismissed or not well received. Your loved one may resent your efforts to be supportive and think that you're being critical or controlling and that you're overstepping your role. Simply put, they may not want or appreciate your input.

Also, your loved one may choose to open up to their therapist, psychiatry provider, or peers rather than you. This can be confusing, and you might even feel jealous (e.g., "But I'm his mom . . . why doesn't he talk to me?"). It can be easier to share personal information with people outside your immediate circle of friends and family, so try to be grateful that your loved one has people they can talk to.

Have there been times when your loved one didn't want your advice or input? If so, describe: _____

_____

_____

What were those times like for you?

How did you manage those situations?

Consider the following tips for times when you feel pushed away:

- Allow yourself to feel all of your emotions—perhaps angry, confused, worried, rejected, powerless, or sad. It hurts when your loved one won't let you in.

- Take care of yourself. Check out appendix B (Activities to Lift Your Spirit) for ideas on self-care strategies.

- Respect your loved one's boundary and give them space (unless they are in crisis—more on managing emergencies in chapter 16).

- Try not to take their limit personally. Remember that their actions may be due to their illness and not a reflection of you or your relationship. Lack of motivation, fatigue, low self-esteem, and problems with attention and follow-through are common among people with a mental illness, all of which can make moving toward goals more challenging.

- Consider that your loved one may lack awareness of their illness or the severity of their mental health problem (termed anosognosia). As we discuss in chapter 13, this difficulty in acknowledging one's illness affects a considerable number of people living with bipolar disorder and schizophrenia and is a common reason that people avoid treatment or stop taking their medications.

- Try to remain available to your loved one and keep lines of communication open. Let them know you respect their choices, and remind them of your love and availability. These messages help them feel comfortable to return when they're ready.

Chapter 7

NAVIGATING THE HEALTH CARE SYSTEM

T HE HEALTH CARE SYSTEM CAN BE challenging to navigate. This chapter examines strategies to support your loved one as they seek treatment for mental illness.

IN THIS CHAPTER, YOU WILL

Consider ways to empower your loved one as they navigate the health care system by

✓ Learning about mental illness

✓ Gaining an understanding of treatment options

✓ Reviewing tips on how to locate mental health professionals as well as screening questions to ask potential providers

✓ Working effectively with the health care team

Note: While this chapter covers some key aspects of interacting with the health care system, subsequent chapters address related topics, including common fears that deter people from seeking help and strategies for talking with your loved one about accessing treatment (chapter 13). Chapter 16 deals specifically with mental health crises, including issues related to suicide, violence, and hospitalizations.

Learning about Mental Illness

Information about mental illness is now readily available to the general public, including facts about causes, risk factors, common symptoms, and treatment options. You can access information by

- Reading blogs, memoirs, and nonfiction books—written by professionals or people with lived experience

- Taking classes and connecting with others through the National Alliance on Mental Illness (NAMI; see details in chapter 3), the Depression and Bipolar Support Alliance (DBSA; see appendices E and F for more details), social media groups, or similar programs

- Watching movies, TED Talks, or other videos

- Listening to podcasts

- Talking with professionals and others with similar experiences

We offer a few points of caution as you seek information:

- Pay attention to the author or source, especially for online materials. Given the lack of quality control on the internet, be cautious about what you read. If the author is affiliated with a university or hospital, the content is more likely to be grounded in science. Some trustworthy sources are included in the Resource List.

- Remember that each person's experience of mental illness is unique. Two people who have been diagnosed with major depression, for example, may have very different sets of symptoms and function quite differently. Your loved one is the expert in their illness.

- Memoirs can be powerful, poignant ways to learn about mental illness. They give a first-hand view of real-life experiences, which can help readers feel validated and less alone. However, these stories can be triggering and distressing, so use caution when reading them.

Gaining Understanding of Treatment Options

In addition to learning about mental illness, it can be helpful to broaden your understanding of different treatment options. Many treatments exist, and they vary in intensity, duration, focus, facilitator, and format. Many people use several modes of treatment simultaneously.

Keep in mind that availability, wait lists, insurance coverage, and access can vary considerably, and options in rural areas may be more limited. When treatments for your loved one are not readily available, you can feel overwhelmed and frustrated. You may become the default health care team . . . but likely without the benefits of professional training, back-up, or time off. During this waiting time, be sure to take good care of yourself.

Treatment Options for Your Loved One

Appendix E (Mental Health Professionals, Services, and Support Groups) describes many common treatment approaches, explains the roles of different mental health professionals, and addresses the benefits of peer support groups. People experiencing mental health concerns benefit from different levels of care depending on their current well-being and needs. Treatment services described in the appendix include

Counseling and testing (psychological services)

Medication management (psychiatry services)

Electroconvulsive therapy (ECT)

"Treatment resistant" therapies

Peer support (also see chapter 6)

Case management

Coaching (supported employment, academic support)

Clubhouse membership (community resource center)

Assertive community treatment (ACT) teams

Partial hospitalization program (PHP) or intensive outpatient program (IOP)

Residential treatment

Short-term stabilization (hospitalization)

Crisis services

Note: Chapter 16 also deals specifically with mental health emergencies, including issues related to suicide, violence, and hospitalizations.

Treatment Options That Target or Include Family Members and Friends

You can support your loved one with their treatment in many ways. Because you have a shared history and likely frequent contact, you have important information regarding their strengths, challenges, and history. You can offer emotional support, help them make progress on their goals, and empower them with their treatment plan. For example, you might encourage them to participate in therapy, exercise regularly, stay connected to family and friends, and keep up with their medications.

You may also participate in treatment services directly, either with your loved one or on your own. Growing research is demonstrating the benefits of involving families in care—for you, your loved one, and your relationship.[42]

For example, couples therapy can offer tools for working on your relationship with your loved one such as managing conflict, working together in dealing with the illness, intimacy, communication, and problem-solving. It's important to select a couples therapist who has specific training and expertise in working with mental illness. Some couples therapy approaches focus on a specific condition, such as Family-Focused Therapy for Bipolar Disorder (FFT) developed by Dr. David Miklowitz, and Cognitive-Behavioral Conjoint Therapy for Post-traumatic Stress Disorder (CBCT for PTSD) created by Drs. Candice Monson and Stephanie Fredman.

Appendix F (Family Education Programs and Support Groups) describes a range of education and treatment programs for friends/family members. Both family educational classes and support groups can offer a safe space to share your experience and receive support from peers and professionals. You can learn skills about managing crises, setting limits, strengthening your relationship, and communicating effectively with your loved one.

Locating Mental Health Professionals

Finding high-quality, culturally-informed mental health care can be very difficult. Here are some strategies you might consider:

- Explore online directories
  - Visit the Substance Abuse and Mental Health Administration (SAMHSA)'s website (www.findtreatment.gov) which has up-to-date information about treatment options (or call their anonymous hotline at 1-800-662-HELP)
  - For therapy and psychiatry, do a free search on the Psychology Today website: www.psychologytoday.com. You can use filters to select providers with specific areas of expertise, such as faith, ethnicity, sexual orientation, etc.

- ○ You may find websites with lists of providers who identify with certain personal characteristics, such as Muslim therapists, Asian counselors, or psychiatrists who identify as LGBTQ+ (or are affirming). These directories vary by location, but an online search may be useful. Examples of specific online therapist directories include: InnoPsych (therapists of color: www.innopsych.com), Asian Mental Health Collective (www.asianmhc.org), National Queer & Trans Therapists of Color Network (www.nqttcn.com), and Latinx Therapy (www.latinxtherapy.com).

- Ask your insurance company what providers are "in network" and what services are covered.

- Contact your local community mental health center or federally qualified health center because many providers accept Medicare or Medicaid. Some centers also offer a sliding scale fee for people without insurance.

- Explore options in your community that provide free or low-cost counseling services such as an Employee Assistance Program (EAP) through your employer, churches/houses of worship, and local colleges or universities (you may call their psychology or psychiatry department and ask if they have a community clinic).

- Ask for personal recommendations from a primary care doctor, family members, friends, clergy/ministers, or local advocacy organizations such as the National Alliance on Mental Illness (NAMI) or the Depression and Bipolar Support Alliance.

Screening Questions to Ask Potential Providers

Mental health providers and treatment programs vary considerably, and sometimes it's hard to know where to start in finding and selecting one. Appendix E (Mental Health Professionals, Services, and Support Groups) describes many treatment options as well as the roles of various mental health professionals. When searching in your community, you may get helpful information from clinic and provider websites, including patient reviews. Some therapists offer a free, brief phone consultation to help you decide if they're a good fit.

Interview prospective providers and programs. Ask about what's important to you. You may consider some of the questions in the following table.

Important: Although all of these questions about selecting mental health professionals are useful, perhaps the most important variable is not something that can be gleaned from a website or recommendation—namely, do you feel like you connect to the provider. It may take a couple visits to figure that out. Listen to your gut. Do you sense that the provider is really listening? That they care about you as a person? That they want to help you? Even if a provider has amazing credentials and years of experience, if you don't feel seen or cared about, try to find someone else.

QUESTIONS ABOUT PROVIDERS AND TREATMENT OPTIONS

Mental Health Provider

Quality and reputation	How long have you been practicing? Could you tell me about your training and credentials?
Trustworthiness	Are you licensed? Are you affiliated with a hospital, organization, or professional group?
Treatment approach	How do you approach treatment? Do you have experience with my concerns? Do you use evidence-based treatments?
Cultural sensitivity and competence	Do you understand my cultural identity and how that shapes my experience of mental illness and health? If unfamiliar with my culture, are you open to learning?

Treatment Programs

Treatment elements	What are the components of treatment, such as medication, therapy, classes, support groups, or wellness activities?
Format	Are services delivered in individual or group formats?
Provider(s)	Who specifically provides the service (professionals or peers)?
Family involvement	Can family members (including children) participate? If so, how?
Secular versus spiritual or religious	Is the treatment secular or based on a particular religious or spiritual approach? Does the treatment draw upon the 12-step model?

Quality of Services

Effectiveness	Do you have any data or research showing that the treatment is helpful?
Potential risks	What are the possible short- and long-term risks of this treatment, if any?

Logistics

Schedule	How long do people typically participate in this treatment? When are services offered—daytime, evening, or weekend?
Setting	Are services offered in person, online, or some hybrid model? Where are services provided?
Cost and insurance coverage	What are the out-of-pocket costs? Does my insurance cover this service? Is pre-authorization needed?
Access	Is there a waiting list? When could I begin?

Now that we have explored the importance of learning about mental illness, reviewed various kinds of treatments, and considered screening questions for selecting a provider, the rest of this chapter focuses on how to work well with your loved one's treatment team.

Working Effectively with the Health Care Team

If interacting with the health care system has been difficult, you're not alone. Navigating the complex array of systems, providers, and insurance issues can be confusing, frustrating, and time consuming. Figuring out your role can also be tricky. Consider the following suggestions.

Attend Appointments Periodically if Your Loved One Agrees

Ask your loved one if it's OK for you to accompany them to some appointments. Doing so shows that you want to help and be involved. Offer to take notes if your loved one is OK with your doing so. Respect that the appointment is for your loved one, not you, so try to be concise and supportive when sharing your concerns.

Mental health visits (especially with psychiatry providers) are often brief, and the doctor or nurse may have many issues that need to be assessed. You might bring a list of questions and updates such as major life changes, concerns about medications or side effects, changes in use of alcohol or drugs, and any safety concerns (regarding self-harm, suicide, violence toward others).

> "My wife and I create a list of questions before she meets with her psychiatrist. She and the doctor do most of the talking, and I take notes (which my wife really appreciates). I think my presence also helps to keep her honest. We have her crisis plan, medication list, and notes from appointments in a 3-ring binder so everything is together and organized."
>
> —A HUSBAND

In addition, you and your loved one may create and keep an up-to-date summary of their well-being. Especially when starting with a new provider, this document can save time and facilitate the treatment process. Topics to include are current diagnosis; medications (doses, name of prescriber); active therapies and names of providers; recent stressors; strengths and areas of life that are going well; progress toward life goals; and questions and concerns.

Remember the story of Alexis and Jasmine from the previous chapter in which Alexis is managing significant anxiety? Jasmine found it very helpful to attend her sister's therapy appointment.

Alexis wanted Jasmine to better understand her depression and anxiety, so she invited her sister to join her one of her therapy sessions. Jasmine was touched and eager to meet the therapist and learn more about her sister.

In the appointment, the therapist explained how avoiding situations that frighten Alexis can actually allow her depression and anxiety to continue and possibly worsen. The therapist honored that Jasmine was trying to be helpful by offering to contact local businesses to display the jewelry. However, part of Alexis' treatment plan was to learn how to manage her anxiety so she can handle these situations on her own. This made a lot of sense to Jasmine, and she appreciated learning other ways to support her sister.

Understand Privacy Laws (and Remember You Always Have the Right to Share Information)

The Health Insurance Portability and Accountability Act of 1996 (HIPAA) is a federal law that created national standards for protecting private health information from being released without the person's consent. The HIPAA Privacy Rule (2002) was issued to implement the HIPAA requirements. States also have their own confidentiality laws, some of which are stricter than federal law.

These laws were created with the intent of protecting patient rights, and people seeking mental health care need to be able to trust and feel safe with their providers. However, the restrictions on communication can be frustrating for family members/friends, and can add to the stigma surrounding mental illness.

The specifics of federal and state laws are beyond the scope of this book, but key points include

- You *always* have the right to share information with your loved one's providers, and keeping in regular communication can be invaluable. For example, you may want the psychiatry provider to know that your husband is not taking his medication or is drinking heavily—and you worry that he is not sharing this information openly. If it's not feasible or appropriate to share this information in your loved one's presence, you can

- ○ Call the clinic and leave a phone message
- ○ Drop off a letter
- ○ Request a brief phone conversation with the provider
- ○ Send a message in the electronic health record (but realize your loved one can access this information as well)

Your loved one may feel angry if you pass this information along to their providers. Although dealing with their distress may be uncomfortable, reassure yourself that you're doing the right thing, especially if there are issues of safety or violence. Health care providers can be most helpful when they have accurate information about what's going on, and you have important observations to share.

- Encourage your loved one to consider signing a Release of Information which makes it much easier for you and the treatment team to talk freely. These forms must be signed for each clinic or health care system and need to be signed every year.

- Other than during times of immediate crisis (suicidal behavior, violence, or threats thereof), mental health professionals cannot give you specific information about your loved one without a signed Release of Information. These rules can be upsetting, especially when you want to know how your loved one is doing. Some health care providers will speak in generalities, such as: "I cannot discuss your wife's specific case, but generally speaking when. . . . , I advise. . . ."

Although navigating the health care system can be overwhelming and frustrating, it may get easier with time. Investing time and energy in learning about mental illness, going to appointments, and forming open relationships with your loved one's providers can pay dividends in the long run, especially during times of crisis.

Part III

STRENGTHENING YOUR RELATIONSHIP WITH YOUR LOVED ONE

Chapter 8

STRENGTHENING YOUR CONNECTION

A CROSS ALL KINDS OF RELATIONSHIPS, people want to be seen, heard, understood, and valued. Those desires are simply part of being human, and your loved one wants these things as well. The way in which your loved one desires or experiences connection may vary depending on their preferences and current wellness, but at the core, we all long to be seen and appreciated.

IN THIS CHAPTER, YOU WILL

Consider three ways of strengthening your connection with your loved one by

✓ Expressing fondness, pride, and gratitude

✓ Offering grace and being patient

✓ Spending quality time together

Expressing Fondness, Pride, and Gratitude

Although much of this book explores challenges you may experience with your loved one, it's equally important to focus on what you enjoy about them and your relationship. Mental illness is just one part of your loved one; it does not totally define them nor your relationship. Although you may play many roles in their well-being, such as care coordinator, counselor, advocate, and more, being able to focus on your role as family member or friend at times can help you strengthen your relationship. Of course, focusing on your connection is likely not feasible when your loved one is especially ill, and the tips in chapter 16 may be useful for you at those times.

Taking time to reflect on the positive aspects of your loved one and your relationship is important, and we encourage you to express these sentiments to them as well. The more specific you can be, the better. Avoid overpraising or trying to flatter them, but share the truth. Remember you may be the only person who offers them encouraging words!

So, take a moment and consider if any of these messages might work for you:

One of my favorite activities to do with you is _____

_____

I love how we can talk about our inside jokes or memories of _____

_____

I'm proud of how hard you're working on _____

_____

Even when things are tough, I know you _____

_____

I love hearing you talk about _____

_____

I'm grateful for _____

_____

Research has documented how the act of seeing and acknowledging the goodness in another human being can be powerful, with clear benefits for both the speaker and recipient. For example, grateful people tend to have better mental and physical health, less burnout, greater happiness, and better overall life satisfaction.[43] Research has found that receivers of genuine expressions of gratitude often view the other person and the relationship in a more positive light.[44] Thus, be it a verbal expression of "thanks," a text message, a letter, an email, a video, or a high five, sharing your gratitude can be a booster shot of positivity for your relationship. It can also strengthen your connection and resilience, helping you manage the challenges as a team.

Offering Grace and Being Patient

In addition to strengthening your bond by expressing gratitude and fondness, you can navigate difficulties in ways that improve your relationship as well. Conflict, misunderstandings, hurt feelings, and disappointment can emerge in all relationships. This section offers a perspective for how you can view and respond to your loved one's behavior in ways that improve your connection. The next two chapters offer additional skills, namely developing effective communication strategies and setting limits.

Although the term "grace" can have a religious or spiritual connotation, it can also have broader applications. Offering grace can be showing kindness, love, or forgiveness when someone hurts or disappoints you. Instead of responding in anger and spiraling into critical, judgmental thinking, grace involves remaining calm, patient, and compassionate.

Offering grace does not mean you don't feel hurt or that you don't hold the other person accountable . . . rather, grace involves responding intentionally with kindness. When you can be patient and calmly look at the situation differently, you can also free yourself of tension and pressure. You might choose to let the issue go, or come back at a later time and approach the other person respectfully.

Messages grounded in grace could sound like

- *My loved one is behaving this way because they have an illness—it's not who they are as a person.*

- *I choose to not take this situation personally. Instead, I will offer them compassion.*

- *It must be hard for my loved one to feel so lonely and confused.*

- *I know my loved one is doing their best in a very difficult situation.*

- *Though I strongly dislike my loved one's choices and behavior, I still love and care about them.*

- *Although I'd really like to talk back to my loved one right now, I'm going to take the high road and take a break. I will try again when both of us are calm.*

- *I wish my loved one would get going on their "to do" list. I could do some of the tasks for them, but I'm working hard to be patient and stay in my lane.*

Offering someone grace can be hard, and you definitely won't succeed every time. When you're struggling, remember how good it felt when someone offered you grace. And, remember the power of giving yourself grace as well. As discussed in chapter 2, offering yourself kindness and self-compassion can be comforting and healing.

Is there an issue you're currently facing in which you would like to offer your loved one grace? If so, describe here: _____

> Importantly, extending grace and patience does not mean tolerating abusive or disrespectful behavior—nor does it mean staying in a relationship that is unhealthy for you or your children. Protecting yourself and making tough decisions are vital for your emotional health. Chapter 10 explores limit setting in detail.

Spending Quality Time Together

One of the simplest yet most meaningful ways to improve a relationship is to spend quality time together. Tiny, kind, connecting moments, especially when repeated over time, can be more meaningful than big events such as a vacation.

When you commit to building your connection, it's important to focus on being together without placing any demands, asking prying questions, or trying to solve problems. It's OK for some of the time to be spent in silence. Just being present may be the most helpful thing you can do (and it takes the pressure off of figuring out what to say!). Also, you may wish to avoid addressing hard topics like money, medications, or other possibly contentious issues. Rather, focus on enjoying each other's company.

Here are some activities you and your loved one might enjoy doing together. Perhaps you already do some of them. See if any others sound appealing, and write in additional ideas that come to mind.

Get Moving Together

- Go on a walk or hike

- Go to the gym or try out a yoga class

- Go for a bike ride

- Play pickleball

- _____

Relax Together

- Read on the deck or in front of the fireplace

- Watch a sporting event

- Cook their favorite meal

- Play cards or a board game

- Do a jigsaw puzzle

- Look through old pictures or videos

- _____

Think Deeply and Learn Together

- Read and discuss a blog, article, or book

- Watch a movie or TV series, and talk about your reactions

- Learn something new together, such as how to cook a new dish

- Take a community education class together

- _____

Go on Mini-Adventures and Enjoy Beauty Together

- Go on a car ride and have a picnic (perhaps get take-out from your loved one's favorite restaurant)

- Go to a museum or local art festival

- Hike at a park. Appreciate the nature that surrounds you—what you hear, see, smell, and feel

- Go to a free concert in the park or a high school/college music concert

- _____

Discuss and Practice Your Values and Beliefs

- Talk about what really matters to you

- Pray or meditate

- Try out a new church or house of worship

- Find ways to serve others, possibly by volunteering

- Give them a chance to be a friend to you—ask for their help. Doing this can offer them opportunities to live out the value of helping others

- _____

We realize this suggestion of spending quality time together may sound overly simplistic. In reality, this can be much more nuanced and complicated. For example, you may have bills to pay, laundry to do, and other responsibilities that are piling up . . . making it hard to dedicate time to your loved one. Also, perhaps you have others in your life who need you, and spending time with them can feel more relaxing.

In addition, we recognize that

- Your loved one may ignore or decline your invitations

- Your loved one may agree but then cancel at the last minute

- You may not know if your loved one enjoyed the activity or felt any better afterwards

- The interaction may not bring the closeness you hoped for

- Your loved one may not thank you for the activity

All of these outcomes can happen. The reality is your loved one may not want to spend time with you—no matter what you suggest. Perhaps they are overwhelmed by their emotions or thoughts; interacting with you would be too anxiety provoking, exhausting, or stressful. They might feel embarrassed or ashamed, fear your judgment, or want to avoid being asked too many questions. Perhaps they're irritated with you and simply need some distance for a while.

Regardless of the reason, it's important to give your loved one space and respect their boundary. Otherwise, your well-intended involvement may be experienced as unhelpful, annoying, and possibly controlling

Depending on the situation and length of time they are withdrawing, you might reach out in gentle ways, such as sending a text message or offering to drop off a home-cooked meal. As challenging as their withdrawal can be, continue making yourself available. Avoid badgering, but remind them that they matter and that you're there for them.

When your loved one is distant, it's understandable that you may feel discouraged, rejected, confused, and hurt. As discussed in chapter 6, it can be painful and worrisome when your loved one doesn't want your support. Your inability to spend time with them may exacerbate your concerns about them. For your own well-being, be sure to stay connected to your own support system and engage in enjoyable activities, either alone or with others.

Simply put, no matter if you are expressing fondness and gratitude, offering grace, or spending time together, you can strengthen your relationship by saying and living out these simple yet profound messages:

I see you.
I believe in you.
I hear you.
I'm safe.
I'm on your team.
I value you.
I love you.

ADAPTED FROM MENNANO[45]

Chapter 9

COMMUNICATION

LEARNING TO COMMUNICATE EFFECTIVELY and keeping open lines of communication with your loved one are two of the best things you can do for your relationship. It takes courage to be honest and vulnerable, and relationships can deepen through sharing. On the other hand, name calling, angry attacks, and the silent treatment can be deeply hurtful. Today's digital world has created more ways to connect, yet has also made communication more complicated.

Communicating with someone living with a mental illness can be especially challenging.

Do you find it difficult to communicate with your loved one? If so, how? _____

_____

_____

Do you communicate differently with them than with other people? If so, how? _____

_____

_____

Are there certain topics that are easy to discuss? _____

_____

_____

What topics tend to be more difficult? _____

_____

_____

✓ Review common communication challenges

✓ Learn five helpful tips about communication, including consideration of the role of culture

✓ Consider specific skills for
  o Sharing your thoughts and feelings
  o Responding to your loved one

✓ Learn about asking for feedback on how to be supportive

Common Communication Challenges

You might struggle when trying to communicate with your loved one for a variety of reasons. Consider the following common scenarios, and check those that you relate to.

When I reach out to my loved one . . .

They get defensive, angry, or overwhelmed:

- *They tell me to leave them alone; I feel so shut out.*

- *They go from 0 to 100 in an instant. They get mad no matter what I say or do.*

- *They get tearful and anxious so easily. I never know what's going to set them off, so it's hard to know what to say. I don't want to hurt them but need to be able to speak my truth.*

- *They ridicule or make fun of me—the sarcasm really hurts. I sometimes wonder why I keep trying . . .*

They don't share their thoughts and feelings:
- *Why won't they let me in and share what's going on? In public, they put on a mask and pretend everything is wonderful, but I know they're really hurting.*

- *Sometimes I wonder if they even care . . . not only do they not talk about their own feelings, but they don't ask me how I'm doing. They seem more interested in videogames than me.*

They struggle to trust me since their trauma:
- *They seem haunted by what happened to them. I get that everything has changed for them, but I'm still here. I want to understand.*

- *They push me away as if I were the enemy. It's like they can't trust me . . . even though I'm not the one who hurt them . . .*

Their symptoms make it hard for us to communicate:
- *It's like I can't reach them . . . They seem distracted and in their own world.*

- *They respond in confusing ways to emotions, such as staring off into space when I share something important.*

- *They are focused on things I can't see or hear—I honestly don't know what to say.*

Other reactions you experience: _____

_____

_____

Look at the items above and circle those that are most difficult. Then, take this space below to describe how you feel in those situations. What's it like for you to reach out but not connect with your loved one—when your attempts are ignored or rejected? How do you cope with those situations? _____

_____

_____

> **Note:** It can be helpful to remind yourself that your loved one's reactions are often related to their illness and are not a reflection of something about you or your relationship. As hard as it can be, try to avoid taking their behavior personally. You may find it helpful to connect with a trusted friend when you feel dismissed or shut out.

Helpful Communication Tips

Although communication can certainly be challenging, you and your loved one can learn skills that make a big difference. In this section, we describe

- General pointers about communication

- Tips for sharing your thoughts and feelings

- Tips for responding to your loved one

We meet Mathias and his parents, Ethan and Rebekah, and see how they handle a tough situation. We first consider a scenario in which their communication doesn't go well (Round One), and then look at interactions where they use more effective communication skills and have a better outcome (Round Two).

General Pointers about Communication

Before looking at specific tips for sharing and responding, let's consider a few general suggestions about communication. Although this book focuses on interacting with a loved one with a mental illness, the skills in this chapter apply to communicating with anyone who is important to you.

1. **Talk to each other in person.** Today's high-tech world allows people to communicate in many ways via a variety of platforms. Digital communication such as texting and instant messages has some advantages, such as the ability to use pictures, memes, emoji, and videos. The asynchronous nature of messaging enables people to send, read, and respond to messages when convenient rather than in real time. Digital messages can also be a simple way to let someone know you're thinking about them.

   However, a lot can get lost or misunderstood in digital communication. Risks may include

   - Missing important parts of the message: Tone of voice, eye contact, gestures, and pauses convey vital information and provide context for words. Digital communication lacks all of these, resulting in the listener only getting a narrow part of the message.

   - Misinterpretation: Is that emoji, meme, or video meant literally? Or is intended to be playful and a joke? Or is it sarcastic? (Sarcasm can be confusing for people with a serious mental illness and is especially hard with digital communication.)

   - Avoidance of vulnerability: Texting may feel easier or emotionally safer than talking in person; some people say things via digital communication they would never say directly.

   Because of these risks, in-person dialogue is usually best for sensitive topics. If physical distance makes getting together impossible, a video chat may be a good option.

2. **Consider cultural influences.** Everyone has their own unique way of communicating, and both our words and nonverbal messages can result in misunderstandings. Different cultures and families can have vastly different communication styles. Culture can involve not only race or ethnicity, but many other variables as well such as socioeconomic status, education, gender identity, sexual orientation, language, physical ability, religion and spirituality, immigration status, veteran or military, and more. These are all broad categories, and considerable individual differences exist within each group.

   As most of the tips in this section are grounded in Western traditions, it's important to consider cultural norms that can affect how you communicate. For example, in some cultures, people tend to limit eye contact and nonverbal feedback such as head nodding. Disagreeing openly can be taboo in cultures where harmony, tolerance, and sacrificing one's own needs for the sake of others are important values. Norms about manners of speech can vary, with some cultures using very straightforward, precise communication with others using more subtle, indirect messages. Expression of strong feelings is discouraged in some cultures where restraint is valued. Thus, consider how culture may affect your communication, and strive to understand and respect differences.

3. **Consider a walk or a drive.** You and your loved one may communicate well when sitting down and making direct eye contact. For some people, however, extended eye contact is uncomfortable. Therefore, consider initiating conversations while you're doing something together, such as going on a drive or a walk. Many people feel more relaxed and freer to talk openly when engaged in an activity.

4. **Try weekly check-ins.** It's easy to avoid talking directly about tough topics because these conversations can be uncomfortable. You might schedule a weekly time for you and your loved one to intentionally connect. You can commit to approaching the check-ins with an open mind, ready to share honestly and listen to each other.

5. **Take a break.** If tempers rise or things are getting nowhere, take a break. Give each other space, and try again later. It's much better to settle down and resume when feeling calmer than to have long arguments, including ones that last late into the night. A specific tool for handling these situations, a Time Out process, is described in chapter 10.

   Now that we have reviewed some general concepts about communication, let's turn to skills for sharing your message and skills for responding to your loved one.

SKILLS FOR SHARING

- **Pick a good time:** When raising a sensitive topic, be considerate of how you are both feeling before starting the conversation.
  - Remember HALT: Avoid bringing up important issues when you or your loved one are Hungry, Angry, Lonely, or Tired.

- **Approach with kindness and optimism:** Instead of thinking about "me" versus "him, her, or them," focus on the two of you working together as a team. For example:
  - *We are two smart people who care about each other. We can figure this out!*
  - *Our relationship is more important to me than this issue.*

- **Use a calm and respectful tone.**
  - Speak in an assertive manner (see chapter 10 for tips on assertive communication).
  - Be careful to avoid a judgmental or patronizing tone of voice.

- **Be brief and stay in the present.**
  - Take time to prepare by thinking through your main message, and then limit your sharing to a few sentences.
  - Although it may be tempting to bring up the past, doing so often complicates situations. Stick to one specific, current situation.

- **Avoid asking a lot of questions.** This can result in your loved one feeling overwhelmed or defensive.

- **Speak about your own feelings.** Rather than using blaming words, focus on your own emotions and requests.
  - Consider "I messages" in which you describe your emotions in a non-attacking style and ask specifically for what you want:

When you . . . , I feel . . .

In the future, I would appreciate . . .

- *When you stay out late and don't check in, I feel worried about you. In the future, I would appreciate if you'd drop me a text so I know you're safe.*

- *When I'm talking to you and you stare at your phone, I feel hurt and ignored. In the future, I would appreciate if you'd please put your phone down when we talk about important stuff.*

> "Listen with the intent to understand, not the intent to reply."
>
> STEPHEN COVEY[46]

SKILLS FOR RESPONDING

- **Listen** with your undivided attention.
  - Look at your loved one to show you are paying attention
  - Minimize distractions: turn off the TV or computer; put phones aside
  - Avoid interrupting or talking about your own similar experiences

- **Ask how you can be helpful** but avoid stepping in to fix the problem or offering solutions.
  - Strive to ask open-ended questions that elicit more information than yes/no answers.
  - Here are some questions you might consider:
    - » *How can I show up for you right now? Do you want me to*
      - *Just listen?*
      - *Offer advice?*
      - *Get involved?*

- **Thank your loved one** for sharing with messages such as
  - *I care about you.*
  - *I want to understand your experience.*
  - *Your feelings matter to me.*

Note: If your loved one is experiencing psychotic symptoms (hallucinations or delusions), avoid debating or trying to convince them to change their beliefs.

Mathias and His Parents

To see some of these communication skills in action, let's see how Mathias and his parents (Ethan and Rebekah) handle a tricky situation. In Round One, their discussion deteriorates quickly, everyone is upset, and relationships are strained. In Round Two, they use some of the skills described in this chapter, and the outcomes are quite different.

Mathias, age 21, is enrolled in a carpentry trade school and has been dating Sarah for six months. He recently moved back in with his folks to save money and spends a lot of time in his bedroom downstairs. He dealt with serious depression while in high school, and found an antidepressant and therapy helpful in improving his mood. In the past, he drank heavily and used marijuana frequently.

When Mathias' parents return home from a long weekend away, they find him asleep on the couch mid-afternoon, wearing the same clothes he had on when they left. Rebekah notices that the pill organizer is full—so Mathias likely didn't take his medication while they were gone. When they go downstairs to put their luggage away, they see the lower level is a mess, with pizza boxes, bags of chips, and empty beer bottles on the floor and coffee table. There is a strong smell of marijuana; Mathias knows the family rule of no pot in the house.

Ethan and Rebekah are furious!

Round One

Ethan finds Mathias half-asleep on the couch, and jostles him to wake up.

Ethan (in a loud, attacking, accusing voice): What did you do while we were gone? The basement is a disaster! I told you not to have a party while we were away—who was here? I sure hope you didn't have your friends from high school over; you know they're a horrible influence! And you know our rule of no pot allowed in our house—ever. Who do you think you are?

Mathias (mumbling): What's going on? Why are you hollering at me? I was sleeping.

> Remember HALT: communication is harder when we're hungry, angry, lonely or tired. Ethan is angry and Mathias is sleepy.

> Remember to approach your loved one with respect, using a quiet, calm tone of voice.

> Avoid repeated questions that can make the listener feel defensive.

> Remember to keep your communication succinct. Your loved one may feel overwhelmed and not respond to any of your questions when you go on and on.

Ethan: Every time we leave, you make a mess. We can't even leave you alone for a few days. You are so disrespectful. You knew we were getting home today—you didn't even have the common courtesy to pick up before we got home. You should be grateful that we let you live here rent free.

> Try to stay in the present. When Ethan refers to "every time," he is making a generalization which can distract from the present situation.
>
> Avoid talking down or judging your loved one.

Mathias: Get off my back. You have no idea what happened this weekend—it was one of the worst weekends of my life.

Ethan (ignoring what Mathias just said): And your mom saw your pill organizer. and it looks like you didn't take your meds while we were gone. How in the world do you think you're going to get better if you don't take your medicine? I just don't know what to do with you.

> Stick to one topic at a time.
>
> Speak about your own feelings rather than using blaming words ("you").

Mathias (yelling while walking out of the room): Leave me alone. You just don't get it.

Mathias goes to his bedroom and slams the door. He refuses to talk for several days and seems more depressed than ever.

Ethan feels horrible about how he talked to Mathias. He doesn't know what to do.

Round Two

Let's replay this conversation and consider how Ethan could have handled it differently. It's absolutely understandable that Ethan and Rebekah would feel angry and disappointed. There's nothing wrong with having those feelings. How they manage and express their emotions can make a big difference. In this round, they choose to offer him grace.

Feeling livid when they see Mathias and the messy basement, Ethan and Rebekah go on a walk. They both vent, sharing their frustration and confusion. They decide to wait until Mathias wakes up to talk to him.

> If you're emotionally overwhelmed, take a break to calm down before approaching your loved one.

> Pick a good time to raise a sensitive topic.

Ethan (in a respectful tone): Hey Mathias. Mom and I had a fun vacation, and we got some great pictures.

Wonder if we could talk about how things went around here this weekend?

Mathias: Well . . . I don't want to talk about it, but OK . . .

Ethan (puts his cell phone away, mutes the television, and sits down): Thanks. I felt pretty upset to find the basement such a mess when we got home. Could you help me understand what happened?

> Minimize distractions and get at the same level.
>
> Thank the other person for being willing to talk.
>
> Express your own feelings rather than accusing.

Mathias: Yeah, well . . . things kinda got out of control, but . . . the worst part was . . . Sarah broke up with me Friday night. I felt like my world ended. It's just so complicated, Dad.

I needed to escape so I invited a couple friends over. They brought a couple other guys I didn't know and . . . well, things spiraled from there.

Ethan: Thanks for telling me—I'm sorry about Sarah. I know you care a lot about her. I understand how you would feel really lousy . . . and I'm sorry you're going through such a hard time.

⟵ Validate the other person's feelings.

Show that you care. Avoid trying to fix.

Mathias: Yeah, Dad, it's awful. I miss her so much. We're still texting, but it's weird. My depression has just gone through the roof.

By the way, um, I'm sorry about the basement. I couldn't turn those other guys away, and they brought the pot. I'm gonna clean up today, and it won't happen again.

Ethan: Thanks, Mathias. Hey, how about if I help you with the basement?

Please let me know if there are other ways I can support you. You know I'm here to listen.

Asking for Feedback on How to Be Supportive

In Round Two of this scenario, Mathias was open with his dad, and Ethan had the opportunity to express support. In reality, sometimes it's hard to know how to communicate that you care. You may sense that your loved one is hurting but not know what to do. You may want them to share their thoughts and feelings, but trying to pry it out of them doesn't work. Continuing to push and ask questions typically backfires, so being patient and offering space may be helpful.

You might consider the following: When your loved one is feeling well, specifically ask what they would like during challenging times, with a question such as

When you . . . , how can I help?

Example: *When you're going through a tough time and being triggered a lot by the past, how can I show up for you? What could I do to be supportive?*

When you're in a really dark place, I don't know how to help. I want to be there, but don't know what to do. Could you think about it and let me know? Or, am I doing something that bothers you?

When you _____ *, how can I help?* _____

_____

_____

_____

_____

Your loved one may not know how to answer your question, and that's OK. They may say "nothing." They may take some time to think about it. Regardless of their answer, asking the question and expressing your desire to help can open a door.

Let's return to Mathias and Ethan:

Two weeks later, Ethan noticed Mathias seemed down and wondered how he was doing with the break-up. Ethan suggested they go on a drive together and was pleasantly surprised when Mathias agreed. After they caught up on their favorite TV series, Ethan asked how he was feeling about Sarah. Mathias shared how much he misses her and how lonely and lost he feels without her. He's gotten back to the gym to lift weights, which helps some, but he knows it's going to take some time.

The relaxed drive gives Ethan the opportunity to ask a question he's had on his mind for a while. He asks Mathias what he could do to be supportive when the depression is bad. Mathias said he wasn't sure but appreciated the question and would think about it. Mathias said that just spending time together is helpful, and he would like his dad to check in with him from time to time. Mathias could tell that his dad really cared and was trying to help . . . and that felt good.

> "The most healing gift you can give to someone in pain is the awareness that you are honestly trying to understand what they are going through, even if you get it wrong."
>
> TREVOR HUDSON[47]

Chapter 10

LIMIT SETTING

ALTHOUGH PEOPLE WE LOVE CAN BE amazing sources of encouragement and comfort, they can also get under our skin like no one else, leaving us feeling irritated, disrespected, angry, or hurt. Navigating upsetting issues is all part of being in a close relationship, and matters can be more challenging when your loved one has a mental illness.

Ignoring these problems over time can result in resentment and distance in your relationship. Therefore, it's helpful to learn how to work together and give feedback in a respectful manner. This kind of open communication can strengthen, instead of damage, your relationship . . . and leave you feeling better about yourself.

IN THIS CHAPTER, YOU WILL

✓ Learn about triggers and setting limits

✓ Consider the challenges in setting limits by
  - Identifying barriers to setting limits
  - Reflecting on managing self-doubt and guilt
  - Identifying consequences of not setting limits

✓ Look within and consider how you want to respond to triggers by
  - Reflecting on your values that can guide you
  - Learning a four-step process for how to thoughtfully respond to triggers (4 Cs)
  - Learning how to do square breathing, a helpful tool to calm your nervous system

✓ Learn skills for how to set limits effectively by
  - Communicating in an assertive manner
  - Using a Time Out process to disengage from escalating conflicts

Common Triggers

When you feel angry, hurt, or disappointed by your loved one's behavior, you may be "triggered." You may have strong feelings and critical thoughts about what they did (or did not do) and why.

What does your loved one do that triggers you? _____

_____

_____

How do you typically respond? _____

_____

_____

How do you feel about yourself afterwards? _____

_____

_____

You may become defensive or verbally aggressive when you feel triggered; at other times, you may withdraw and shut down. These reactions can become almost automatic—you act without thinking about how you want to respond. You may feel guilty later for how you handled the situation and wish you could take back your hurtful words or behavior.

Your power lies in your ability to **choose** *how to respond to things that trigger you.*

You may decide to ignore some triggering behaviors, and picking your battles is a wise strategy. However, everyday small conflicts can build up and create bitterness and tension over time. Other behaviors may be so distressing (or even dangerous) that you decide to set a clear limit.

Setting Limits

Limit setting starts with *figuring out what you want and need* in your relationship. It can be asking yourself these questions: *What is acceptable? What's OK and what's not OK? What needs to change for my own well-being?*

It can also be *setting parameters on your time and energy.* You may continually re-evaluate what feels like an "appropriate" level of involvement with your loved one, while keeping some distance for your own health. For example, you may derive a lot of fun and sense of community from your tennis league, so Tuesday night matches are a priority. Even when things are tough with your loved one, you maintain this limit and get out to the tennis court.

Having defined the limit, you draw *a clear line* and communicate that to your loved one (if appropriate). For example, you may set a limit that everyone in the house will participate in cleaning shared spaces. You may communicate that it's not OK to smoke in the house, to raise your voice, or to call names during conflict.

It's important to communicate the limit during a calm time, not in the middle of a conflict. Oftentimes limits need to be clarified and repeated over time. Quite commonly the other person may "test" the limit, so it's important to be clear and consistent. Try to avoid setting a limit you're not able to follow through on . . . not an easy task for sure.

Limit setting is a key skill in maintaining your wellness and compassion. Although sticking with limits can be hard, they preserve your energy in the long run, allowing you take care of yourself and support your loved one over time.

The rest of this chapter is organized into three sections:

- Challenges in setting limits

- Looking within and considering how you want to respond to triggers

- Learning skills for how to set limits effectively

Challenges in Setting Limits

Identifying Barriers to Setting Limits

Although the idea of setting limits sounds easy, actually creating and sticking to them can be hard. You may struggle with balancing empathy for your loved one's mental health problems with your need to set limits for your own well-being.

Consider the following challenges that many family members and friends face when setting limits. Check those that you relate to.

_____ **Fear of being selfish:** *Is it even OK to ask? Am I putting my needs before theirs?*

_____ **Uncertainty and self-doubt:** *Is this limit reasonable? Am I doing the right thing?*

_____ **Difficulty expressing my needs:** *How would I even bring it up?*

_____ **Feeling burned out:** *Do I have the energy to stick with the limit?*

_____ **Guilt:** *But maybe I shouldn't because . . . ?*

_____ **Fear of others' judgment:** *Will other people look down on me?*

_____ **Risk of causing tension in our relationship:** *Is it worth it?*

_____ **Risk of my loved one's anger or violence:** *Could it be risky or dangerous?*
(If this is a concern, please see chapter 16 on dealing with threats or violent behavior).

_____ **Others:** _____

> "Ever since my brother's serious car accident,
> he's basically stopped helping out with our parents.
> He used to do their grocery shopping and take them
> to church, but now he cancels more often than not.
> I know he's struggling emotionally, but our folks need
> him . . . and, actually I need him, too. Whenever I
> bring it up, he gets defensive and angry—I just don't
> know how to talk to him. I feel guilty for even asking,
> but I just can't do it all on my own . . ."
>
> **—A SISTER**

Dealing with Self-Doubt and Guilt: Remember Why You're Setting Limits

Although all of these barriers can be significant, self-doubt and guilt can be especially sneaky and subtle. If these feelings creep up, remind yourself why you're setting the limit. Although your mind may quickly agree with the following pointers, convincing your heart can take time. Circle the two or three messages that resonate with you now:

- *I deserve to be treated with respect; my feelings and needs are just as important as theirs.*

- *Even though this is hard, I know it's the right thing to do.*

- *It's not my responsibility to meet my loved one's needs all of the time (nor is it helpful for them or our relationship).*

- *It's OK to disappoint my loved one sometimes.*

- *I can be more patient and supportive after I've taken time for myself.*

- *I am not my loved one's therapist. I'm not trained to do so, and it's not my job.*

- *Other people in my life need me as well. I can't give my loved one all my time and energy—that's not fair to everyone else.*

- Others: _____

  _____

  _____

You may find it helpful to review these messages when self-doubt or guilt arise. You could put the messages on sticky notes or in your phone as reminders. Initially, setting limits can be awkward and challenging; however, doing so usually gets easier with practice. It's important to speak your truth.

Consequences of Not Setting Limits

If you relate to some of the barriers to setting limits, you know how difficult it can be. It's true that sticking with them can be exhausting, and choosing the path of least resistance may be attractive. And sometimes, that's definitely OK. However, what is the cost of doing so over time?

Consider the examples on page 120 of possible fallout for not setting or sticking with limits. Feel free to write in others that come to mind for you.

Like with other diseases such as asthma, mental illness is a long-term condition for some people. Due to the cyclical nature of mental illness, remember that supporting your loved one is often a "marathon," not a "sprint." Clear and consistent limits can help you and your relationship over time.

Now that we've explored the importance of setting limits, let's examine how to set limits in a way that is consistent with your values.

> "We once had to get a restraining order for our daughter. I told her we hated to do it, but had to because of how she was acting toward us. We removed it three months later when she was sober, and we were all relieved."
>
> —A MOM

Possible Consequences of Not Setting Limits

Your Feelings

- Anxiety or self-doubt
- Sadness or depression
- Feel used, taken advantage of, and disrespected
- Feel stuck or powerless
- _____
- _____

Your Feelings toward Your Loved One

- Resentment or anger
- Impatience
- Less empathy for them
- Worry that you are enabling them
- _____
- _____

Your Health and Well-being

- More likely to get physically sick
- Exhaustion—physical, social, spiritual, mental
- Increase in drinking, use of drugs, or other addictive behavior
- Struggle to keep up with other responsibilities (parenting, work)
- _____
- _____

Your Relationships

- Other relationships are neglected
- Guilt for how your loved one's behavior impacts others
- Unsure what to say to others
- Redirecting your anger onto others
- _____
- _____

Looking Within and Considering How You Want to Respond to Triggers

Before considering how to respond to your loved one when their behavior is triggering, it's helpful to look within. Think about how **you** want to show up in this relationship. People feel better about themselves and usually have happier relationships when they act in ways that are consistent with their values.

Reflecting on Your Values

Describe the kind of person you want to be in this relationship. What traits or qualities do you try to live out? _____

_____

How would you like your loved one to describe you? _____

_____

What helps you behave in ways that are consistent with these values? _____

_____

What makes it hard to live according to your values? _____

_____

> "Even when it's hard, I try to be patient, supportive, and empowering of my son. He knows I always have his back . . . no matter what."
>
> —A DAD

As we now consider how to handle triggers, remember the core values you identified above. They can help anchor and guide you in choosing how to respond to difficult behavior.

Responding to Triggering Situations: The 4 Cs

This four-step process can help you respond to triggering situations in an intentional manner rather than reacting out of pure emotion.

The steps include

1. Catch

2. Calm

3. Challenge

4. Choose compassion and change

In this section, we describe the tasks associated with each step. Then, we offer examples of how to use the process in several situations.

STEP ONE: CATCH

The first step involves catching yourself when you're experiencing a reaction to an event or situation. You may notice changes in your body that indicate you're upset, such as muscle tension, sweating, flushed face, clenched jaw, or rapid breathing.

As you check in with yourself, pay attention to your reactions. There's no need to judge them or act on them—just notice and honor your

- Feelings

- Thoughts

- Impulse about how to respond (What's my gut reaction? What's my instinct telling me to do or say?)

STEP TWO: CALM

Take a moment to pause before responding. You may visualize a stop sign or say the word "stop" to yourself. Then, do something that calms your spirit. Taking this time helps you feel in control and able to make a choice about how you want to *respond* rather than *react*.

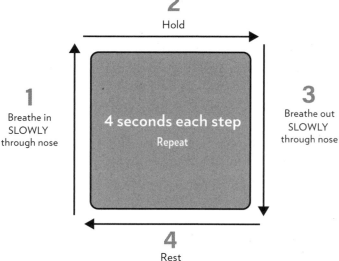

The Square Breathing technique is a useful tool to regulate your nervous system, lower your blood pressure, and help you feel relaxed and calm. It's also useful for insomnia.

2 Hold

1 Breathe in SLOWLY through nose

4 seconds each step Repeat

3 Breathe out SLOWLY through nose

4 Rest

The calming activity does not need to last long, but is something you do intentionally to "press the pause button" before acting. Many people find square breathing (see figure), going on a walk, counting to 10, stretching, or playing with a pet to be grounding and calming.

STEP THREE: CHALLENGE

Now that you have observed and honored your feelings, thoughts, and gut reaction ("catch"), and taken time to calm your nervous system ("calm"), it's time to move to the next step, namely "challenge."

To avoid being driven by your automatic thoughts and strong emotions, approach the situation with openness and curiosity. Instead of jumping into a judgmental mindset and responding impulsively, try to step back a bit and look at the situation objectively. How can you show up in a way that is consistent with your values? As we discussed in chapter 8, how might I offer my loved one grace?

Remember that you and your loved one are two smart people and that you've worked through difficult issues together in the past. You are a team. Your loved one is not the enemy! Approaching the situation with an optimistic attitude can make a big difference.

With that hopeful, open mindset, consider these questions:

1. What kind of a person do you want to be right now?
   o *How can I act in a way that aligns with my values?*
   o *How can I balance supporting my loved one with taking care of myself?*

2. What may be underneath or causing your loved one's behavior?
   o *What might their behavior be trying to tell me?*
   o *Is this a time to show empathy for their struggle with mental illness?*
   o *Could I choose to give my loved one the benefit of the doubt, believing they are doing their best and offering them grace?*

3. What's more important here—being right or your relationship?
   o *Is it worth the energy to address this issue?*
   o *Is this reflecting something else going on in our relationship that needs to be addressed?*

Taking this time to challenge yourself prepares you for the final step.

STEP FOUR: CHOOSE COMPASSION AND CHANGE

Hopefully checking in with yourself during the "challenge" step offered you a new perspective, and you are ready to "choose compassion and change." Importantly, you may decide to do nothing at all—that is definitely a choice. That doesn't mean the issue is not bothersome; it means that you are simply not going to address it at this time. Rather than discussing it with your loved one, you may agree to disagree, ignore the behavior, distract yourself, take a break, decide to deal with it later, or even use humor and make a joke.

If you do choose to respond to your loved one, strive for a compassionate approach, which can be reflected in your words, eye contact, and tone of voice (remember the skills from chapter 9 on Communication). You can be grounded in compassion by believing your loved one is doing their best and by approaching them as a kind friend rather than as a critical judge. It may help to think about how you'd like someone to give you feedback and then use that manner in talking with your loved one.

	CATCH MYSELF		
Triggering event	My feelings	My thoughts	My usual behavior
Partner is emotionally distant and says he needs space.	Hurt, rejected	If you won't be there for me, I won't show up for you either.	Withdraw and dismiss
Sister cancelled our plans for a girls' night out three times in a row!	Confused, hurt, sad, angry	What did I do wrong? Doesn't she like spending time with me?	Take it personally
Daughter ends a heated discussion mid-stream and leaves the room.	Angry, ignored, dismissed	Don't you dare walk away— we need to discuss this now!	Follow her and push her to continue the conversation
My fiancé is so negative; he criticizes me for every little thing	Angry	Get off my back! I've had it . . . you are so negative!	Attack and criticize him in return

There is no guarantee that your new approach will produce the outcome you desire. We cannot control how others will respond. However, you've taken the time and energy to reflect and prepare, have made a decision that aligns with your values, and have approached your loved one with respect and kindness.

Note: *If your loved one responds in an abusive manner, remember that mental illness and PTSD should never be used as an excuse for mistreatment. Attacking, controlling, or shaming behavior is never OK. It is essential to hold your loved one accountable for their behavior, especially if it's repeated, hurtful, or in any way abusive. If you ever feel unsafe, please see the information provided in chapter 16 on managing crises.*

Now let's apply the 4Cs to several common situations by using the chart below:

CALM	CHALLENGE MYSELF	CHOOSE COMPASSION AND CHANGE
	New thought	**New behavior**
🙂	I know his depression is bad right now . . . I believe he's doing his best.	I can give space and be willing to be present when he is ready. In the meanwhile, I have others who can support me.
🙂	Maybe this has nothing to do with me! I know she manages a lot of anxiety. I want to be a supportive sister.	Gently check in with my sister. Try to understand how she's doing. Share my feelings about the cancellations (and don't reschedule until she can commit to coming).
🙂	Maybe my daughter is flooded. Perhaps she is taking a break to calm down because she knows she cannot communicate well now. She doesn't want to say something to hurt me.	I'll give her space and we can continue tomorrow when we're calm. I want her to know I respect her boundaries.
🙂	His criticism doesn't feel good. Maybe he's stressed with all the wedding planning, but it's not OK for him to take it out on me.	I respectfully let him know how I feel . . . and ask him to lift me up rather than put me down.

Now we invite you to think of situations that trigger you and work through the 4Cs process.

Although conflict is inevitable in all relationships, it's how you choose to respond that matters. Learning and practicing the 4Cs take time and energy, but doing so can be a solid investment in your relationship.

	CATCH MYSELF		
Triggering event	My feelings	My thoughts	My usual behavior

CALM	CHALLENGE MYSELF	CHOOSE COMPASSION AND CHANGE
	New thought	New behavior

Skills for How to Set Limits Effectively

Now that you've taken time to think about how to respond to a trigger, you're ready to take action in setting the limit. This section teaches two relevant skills:

- Assertive communication

- A Time Out strategy for dealing with escalating conflicts

Assertive Communication

When you approach your loved one about the limit you are setting, it's helpful to use the communication skills addressed in chapter 9 such as using a respectful and calm tone of voice, speaking succinctly and from your experience and feelings, and using non-blaming language.

Let's look at three different kinds of communication:

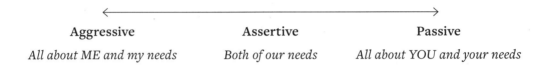

Aggressive	Assertive	Passive
All about ME and my needs	*Both of our needs*	*All about YOU and your needs*

When you are assertive, you honestly, respectfully, and directly express your feelings and wishes. Rather than being aggressive (demanding in a disrespectful manner and focusing only on your own needs) or passive (not expressing your feelings or standing up for yourself), an assertive approach usually has better outcomes.

Examples of these three types:

Aggressive communication: *I can't believe you stopped taking your meds! Do you want to end up in the hospital again? You know what that does to the kids and me . . .*

Assertive communication: *I noticed the pills for the last week are still in your pill organizer. I worry when I see that and would like to understand. I wonder if we could discuss how you feel about your medicines.*

Passive communication: Say nothing

Assertive communication often results in

- You being clear about your limits—what you are and are not willing to do

- You feeling better about yourself and your relationship

- Your connection with your loved one remaining strong or perhaps even growing

- Your loved one feeling respected (rather than judged or attacked)

- Your loved one being able to hear you without feeling a need to defend

Assertive communication works best when you focus on one topic at a time. When your loved one feels overwhelmed by too many requests, they may resent you and push back altogether. Therefore, prioritize what is most important.

Respectful and appropriate communication can vary considerably across cultures. Open disagreement is avoided in some cultures, and people use more indirect messages. Norms about nonverbal communication such as how emotions are expressed, tone of voice, and amount of physical distance between people can also differ. Therefore, consider how your cultural background and that of your loved one may affect how to best express yourself in an assertive manner.

As you've read through this chapter, perhaps a limit has come to mind that you want to set. Consider if you're ready to take action:

What limit might you be ready to set now? _____

_____

_____

What do you need to do to prepare? _____

_____

_____

How could you express it in an assertive manner? _____

_____

_____

What support might you need? Where do you get strength to speak your truth and stick to it? _____

_____

_____

What might get in the way? How could you manage possible obstacles? _____

_____

_____

The Time Out Process

A Time Out is another kind of limit that is useful when arguments start to spiral out of control. Because all relationships have conflict, the goal is not to eliminate differing opinions or disagreements. Rather, it's important to learn how to take a break from these conflicts and come back later to respectfully work through differences.

Research by psychologist Dr. John Gottman has found that human beings simply cannot think or communicate clearly when overwhelmed by strong emotions.[48] Stress hormones surge throughout the body, and tunnel vision can set in. We can't express ourselves clearly and may repeat the same message over and over, sometimes getting louder and more forceful. Also, we can't listen and process new information effectively, which prevents us from understanding other perspectives. Furthermore, we sometimes say or do things that we later regret. When arguments escalate and nothing gets resolved, we can feel bitter, defeated, and discouraged.

Therefore, to prevent arguments from spiraling, it may be helpful for you and your loved one to develop a Time Out process. This skill is far different from the parenting strategy of putting a child in time out; with adults, both members create a process to stop conflicts from spinning out of control.

It's important that you and your loved one discuss and agree to this process during a calm time. You may define a phrase (such as "Time Out") to communicate that you're using this skill.

STEPS IN THE TIME OUT PROCESS

1. Either person can call a Time Out if a discussion is starting to feel intense.
   - It's your responsibility to call it for yourself. Don't tell the other person to "go take a Time Out."
   - Call the Time Out when you first "catch" yourself feeling triggered or sensing the conflict is escalating. It's much easier to take a break early in a conflict before the situation gets heated.

2. The person who called the Time Out physically removes themselves from the room.

3. The discussion ends immediately with no last words on either part.

4. The other person does not follow and does not make any contact (such as texting, calling, emailing, social media posts).

5. During the Time Out
   - Don't obsess about how angry you are, who is right or wrong, or how you can continue your attack later.
   - Do something relaxing such as a walk, meditation, or listening to music.
   - Consider the other person's feelings and possible solutions to the problem.

6. The person who called the Time Out approaches the other person with kindness
   - Return within a few hours of the Time Out but definitely within 24 hours.
   - You may apologize for your part.
   - Start the conversation with a hopeful tone. (*"Let's try this again"* or *"We can do better this time."*)
   - If tempers rise again, take another Time Out.

Like with any new skill, the Time Out process requires practice and commitment from both parties. It may feel awkward at first but gets easier over time. When both members follow the process, arguments are less likely to escalate, thereby protecting the relationship from harm.

Chapter 11

INTIMATE RELATIONSHIPS

U NLIKE THE REST OF THIS BOOK, chapters 11 and 12 focus specifically on intimate partnerships. This chapter explores how mental illness can impact couples and how to strengthen your bond, and chapter 12 addresses parenting with a partner who has a mental illness.

Although intimate relationships can be a source of tremendous meaning and joy, they can also be a lot of work. Couples must negotiate many issues together—finances, communication, chores, intimacy, parenting, and more. When one or both partners live with a mental illness, working together can be more complex and challenging.

IN THIS CHAPTER, YOU WILL

✓ Identify aspects of your relationship that are going well

✓ Identify aspects of your relationship that are challenging

✓ Reflect on coping with uncertainty

✓ Learn specific ways to strengthen your relationship

✓ Consider a few thoughts about physical intimacy

Aspects of Your Relationship
That Are Going Well

Let's start by thinking about what is working in your relationship. Take a moment to consider:

What is going well in your relationship with your partner? _____

_____

_____

What do the two of you do well together? (For example, you may love to travel, engage in meaningful spiritual or religious activities, manage money effectively, or have enjoyable physical intimacy.) _____

_____

_____

In addition to doing activities together, friendship is an important part of close relationships. This may involve listening, being loyal and trustworthy, laughing and enjoying inside jokes, showing affection, and comforting during hard times.

How do you show your partner that you care? _____

_____

_____

How is your partner a good friend to you? _____

_____

_____

Aspects of Your Relationship
That Are Challenging

The fact that half of all marriages in the United States end in divorce reflects the reality that intimate relationships are difficult. With each partner bringing their own life experiences, needs, and perspectives, finding ways to work together can be a challenge. Some differences may be small and easy to manage (for example, what really is the right way to put the toilet paper on the dispenser?), whereas other issues may involve deeply held beliefs, cultural differences, and core values.

When mental illness in one or both partners is added to the mix, relationships can be even more complex. You may feel overwhelmed by not only supporting your partner, but also managing the household, financial issues, parenting responsibilities, and social activities. Finances may be strained if your partner is unable to work consistently, and you may be the primary breadwinner. Given all this, it makes sense that you feel resentful and angry at times with your partner.

Especially when things are tough, it's understandable if you think about a separation or getting a divorce. There are no right or wrong decisions here. Every relationship involves some compromise, and figuring out what you want for your future can be painful. You may also struggle with feelings of guilt and responsibility when contemplating leaving the relationship and how it would impact your partner's mental health. So many things to consider . . . with no easy answers.

The following lists describe issues that are challenging for many couples. Those in the left column apply to all couples, while the topics in the right column are specific to couples managing mental illness. Circle the issues that create conflict or tension in your relationship.

COMMON ISSUES IN MANY RELATIONSHIPS

Alcohol or drug use

Angry outbursts or violence

Communication

Falling out of love

Household chores

Jealousy or infidelity

Lack of quality time together

Money

Parenting

Resentment at being told
 what to do

Sex

Social media use

Trust

Withdrawal from family
 or social activities

Working too much

ADDITIONAL ISSUES FOR COUPLES MANAGING A MENTAL ILLNESS

Denying (or lacking insight into)
 the illness

Guilt or shame at inability to be
 an equal partner in running
 the house or family

Hygiene (showering, changing clothes)

Participating in therapy

Partner's helicoptering
 (over-involvement in treatment)

Taking medications regularly

Threats of self-harm or suicide

Uncertainty if a behavior is due
 to the illness, personality,
 or relationship problems

What and how much to tell others

Next, looking at the items you circled, write about a few of them that are especially difficult right now. Consider this example:

Topic: Getting therapy + What and how much to tell others

My experience: *When we were dating, my partner had intense nightmares, bad anxiety in groups, and a lot of rage. She simply refused to go to parties or holiday gatherings and blew up if I pushed the issue. She seemed haunted by her combat tour in Afghanistan, but neither of us understood what was going on. I nagged her to go to the VA to get help for months, and she resented my telling her what to do. She insisted on keeping everything private, which was hard for me because I needed support. Shortly after we got married, she sought therapy and was formally diagnosed with post-traumatic stress disorder (PTSD). Although hearing that diagnosis was upsetting, knowing what was going on and that treatment was available gave us hope. We still struggle with her social anxiety and worry about others' judgment but are able to talk more openly now.*

Now reflect on a couple of difficult issues for you:

Topic: _____

My experience: _____
_____
_____
_____

Topic: _____

My experience: _____
_____
_____

Coping with Uncertainty: When You Don't Know What to Do

There are probably times when you sense something is going on with your loved one, but you don't know what. Perhaps you aren't sure how to raise your concern. You may fear saying the wrong thing and have no idea how to help. You might worry that your loved one is having severe symptoms or heading for a relapse.

Consider a common pattern between Tessa and her husband, Bashiir, in this diagram. Tessa lives with depression with psychosis; she hears voices when her depression is severe. Lately, she's been spending about 20 hours per day in her bedroom and has worn the same bathrobe for weeks. Bashiir is pretty worried.

Tessa has been feeling more depressed lately.

When she feels overwhelmed, she retreats to her bedroom, takes a nap, or scrolls social media. She doesn't want to talk to anybody. She knows Bashiir can take her withdrawal personally, but she doesn't have the energy to reassure him.

Bashiir feels confused, hurt, and shut out.

Is it me?
What did I do wrong?
Why is she avoiding me?

**Bashiir wonders . . .
what should I do?**

Try to get her to talk?

I know all couples deal with stuff, but I'm worried. I don't know what's going in. I want to ask her how she's feeling, but am afraid of her reaction. She can be so explosive when she feels criticized. I feel so alone and distant from her when this happens.

Give her space?

Maybe she's overwhelmed and not able to talk. If I encourage her to open up, she may feel worse and retreat even more. I sure don't want that. I wonder if she's hearing voices again . . .

This situation between Tessa and Bashiir is common and definitely not easy. Bashiir cannot read her mind, and Tessa isn't in a place to share her feelings. Couples therapy can help you both find ways to honestly communicate your needs and feelings, talk about how symptoms impact both of you, and then respect each other's wishes. Learning and practicing these skills can bring you closer and help you navigate other challenges that arise. Be sure to find a couples therapist who has expertise in working with the mental illness your loved one experiences.

Strengthening Your Relationship

Working on your relationship requires a lot of time, energy, and patience. It's important to try to prevent the mental illness from consuming or defining the relationship. The illness is just one part of what the two of you manage. Nurturing and growing other parts of your relationship is vital.

Many of the skills described in earlier chapters are important building blocks for couples. Let's review some key points that apply to intimate relationships.

Remember you can only change yourself (chapter 5):
- Work to accept the losses associated with mental illness, understanding that some aspects of your relationship may never be the way you would like

- Focus on what is under your control . . . rather than what is not

- Remember you cannot change your partner

Focus on your partner's strengths (chapter 6):
- Pay attention to what you appreciate about your partner

- Regularly remind your partner what you love/admire about them

Work to strengthen your connection with your partner (chapter 8):
- Regularly express how you're proud of your partner

- Share your gratitude for what they bring to your life

- Consider offering grace when a challenge arises

- Spend quality time together

Approach communication with kindness (chapter 9):

- Be optimistic (*"We can do this!"*)

- Sprinkle in respectful humor when appropriate

- Offer the gift of listening without judging, fixing, or interrupting

- Be respectful (words, tone, body language)

- Take a break if things get heated

- Ask your partner how you can be supportive

- Remember you're a team of two smart people who care about each other (rather than enemies trying to win a debate)

- Release your need to be "right" and strive to compromise

Although intimate partnerships have a lot in common with close friendships and other family relationships, some aspects are different. The rest of this chapter focuses on a crucial part of intimate relationships, namely the "glue" or bond that keeps you connected. Knowing your partner is there for you can offer strength during the rough patches in life. In relationships with a strong bond, you know your partner "has your back," and you can count on them.

Glue is a lot different from sticky notes that easily peel away. Relationships that are like sticky notes may look strong and secure on the outside, but they don't stay connected when difficult times arise—partners grow apart or the relationship ends.

So, how do you strengthen the bond in your relationship? Unlike Elmer's® glue where you can use a blow dryer to speed up the bonding process, there's no "blow dryer" for relationships. There's also no fast-forward button. Also, unlike Elmer's glue, which usually requires just a few drops to stick, emotional connection in couples requires ongoing application of love and attention by both members.

Couples can connect and feel close to each other in many ways. You might reflect on what you used to do together. How did you build a close bond early in your relationship?

Turn back to chapter 6 to review some general activities you enjoy doing with your partner. Next, consider the following couple-focused ideas that can strengthen the bond in your partnership.

Demonstrate That You Are Trustworthy
- Keep your commitments: If you say you're going to do something, follow through

- Be loyal and keep each other's secrets

Reach Out and Touch (See Note Below)
- Remember that little things matter—a hug, pat on the back, holding hands, or sitting next to each other on the couch

- Give each other a massage or get a couple's massage

- Ask specifically for what you want or enjoy (rather than what you don't want)

- Be gentle and avoid criticizing your partner

Open Your Heart
- Share your feelings and risk being vulnerable

- Write a love letter

- Listen without judgment

- Send a funny or sweet text message, just to say that you're thinking of them

- Talk about your hopes and dreams for the future

- Tell your partner what you really love about them

- Support and encourage your partner in working toward their goals ("How can I help?")

Seek Professional Help or Resources
- Consider couples therapy (be sure the therapist has specific expertise in treating mental illness)

- Explore talking with clergy or a religious/spiritual leader

- Check out self-help books for couples (Drs. John Gottman and Susan Johnson are authors we especially recommend)

A Few Notes about Physical Intimacy

Physical intimacy can be a powerful way for couples to strengthen and maintain their bond with one another. Many aspects of sexual intimacy can be impacted by mental illness. For example, people experiencing mania (the energetic, happy phase of bipolar disorder) may have more interest in sex than usual and may want to take more risks. On the other hand, depression can involve a decrease or total loss of interest in sexual activity. All of these changes can stem from the mental illness itself, the side effects of medication, and other things going on in the relationship. Some medications (especially some for depression) can both decrease interest in sex and interfere with sexual functioning.

As discussed in chapter 5, changes in intimacy can be a loss for couples managing mental illness. You both may miss the physical and emotional connection you once had, and you may feel distant from each other. As a partner, you may take it personally if your loved one avoids sex or has difficulty enjoying physical intimacy—when, in fact, it may have nothing to do with you or your relationship. Furthermore, talking about sex (with partners, doctors, and therapists) can be uncomfortable, often resulting in couples (and doctors!) avoiding the topic altogether and thus nothing changing.

If you and your partner want to work on your sexual intimacy, you might

- Talk to your primary care provider to see if there may be any physical reasons for the change in interest or ability to enjoy sex, such as medications or other health issues

- Talk to your psychiatry provider to explore options for mental health medications (some may have fewer sexual side effects)

- Explore a variety of ways of creating intimacy as a couple: work to communicate how you can express love to each other, both physically and emotionally, and remember that small regular acts of kindness can go a long way

- Find a couples therapist (or sex therapist) to gain tools and skills for exploring sexual issues in your relationship

Chapter 12

PARENTING WITH A PARTNER WHO HAS A MENTAL ILLNESS OR HAS EXPERIENCED TRAUMA

ALTHOUGH HAVING CHILDREN CAN OFFER a sense of unparalleled feelings of love, anyone who has kids will tell you that being a parent is hard. From dealing with sleepless nights during infancy, to tantrums of preschoolers, to hormones of teenagers, to boomerang kids who return home as adults . . . parenting can be exhausting. Kids don't come with instruction manuals, and it's easy to feel uncertain and overwhelmed.

While it may look like some people have easy, low-stress lives, all families face difficulties. Whenever something significant happens in a family, everyone is affected. Both joyful events (such as the birth of a baby) and challenges (such as loss of a job) can disrupt family life. Roles, responsibilities, routines, and relationships can change.

In the same way, mental illness and trauma can have ripple effects on everyone in the family. The impacts may change over time, and hopefully it gets easier with improved understanding, communication, and treatment. However, because mental illness often goes in cycles, you may live in fear, wondering when a tough spell might be around the corner. This chapter explores how the experience of parenting, as well as the children themselves, can be affected when your partner has a mental illness or has experienced trauma.

IN THIS CHAPTER, YOU WILL

✓ Consider your partner's experience of being a parent

✓ Reflect on your experience of parenting as a team

✓ Learn about common impacts of parental mental illness on kids

✓ Consider eight ways to support your kids and help them cope

✓ Read about resources for your family and children

Your Partner's Experience of Being a Parent

Let's first consider your partner's experience. If your loved one's mental illness had emerged prior to having children, you may have struggled with decisions about becoming parents. Perhaps you balanced your desire to be parents with understandable worries such as the potential risks of psychiatric medications during pregnancy and nursing, how the stresses of children may affect your partner's mental health and parenting capacity, and the fear of your children developing a mental illness.

It's important to note that many people living with a mental illness are dedicated, compassionate, skilled parents. The desire to be an effective, emotionally available parent can motivate people to take care of their mental health and participate in treatment.

Let's think about your family for a moment:

What are your partner's strengths as a parent? What do they do well? _____

_____

_____

What do your kids especially enjoy doing with their parent? _____

_____

_____

Have you let your partner know that you notice and appreciate these strengths and their commitment to parenting? _____

_____

_____

It's also true that mental illness can zap energy and resources, which can be particularly challenging for parents. Here are some ways that parenting can be harder:

- With depression
  - Sadness and exhaustion can make it hard to get up early and prepare your kids for school.

- With mania (phase of bipolar disorder involving very high levels of energy, activity, or mood)
  - Irritability and agitation can make it hard to relax and be patient with your children.

- With trauma survivors or those who have post-traumatic stress disorder
  - The tendency to startle easily at loud noises and discomfort in crowds can make going to a noisy gym for your daughter's basketball game nearly impossible.

- With panic attacks
  - Anxiety in social situations (and fear of the next attack) can make going to the kids' school holiday concert just too daunting.

- With psychosis
  - Hearing voices can make it hard to be present with everyday routines such as reading books with your kids.

Bottom line: mental illness can make it hard for your partner to be the kind of parent they want to be. They may be overwhelmed and quite critical of themselves. They may worry how they can take care of their children when they sometimes struggle to take care of themselves. Further, their guilt and shame around parenting difficulties can damage their self-esteem and worsen their symptoms.

Has your partner's mental illness or past trauma impacted how they parent? If so, how?

_____

_____

_____

What's especially hard for your partner to do with your kids? _____

_____

_____

What helps your partner to stay present and engaged with your children? _____

_____

_____

Now that we have considered your partner's experience, let's look at what it's like for you to work together as parents.

Your Experience of Parenting as a Team

Raising children together as a couple can be a source of tremendous happiness and connection. Sharing the joys of seeing your child take their first steps, graduate from high school, or get that first job can be delightful. However, it's also a lot of work! Parenting involves tremendous responsibility in caring for your children, resulting in less time for you as a couple. Also, you and your partner may disagree about how to raise and discipline your kids, which can create conflicts.

Parenting as a team in the presence of mental illness can be especially challenging. When your loved one is struggling emotionally, they may be less able to engage with the children and co-parent with you. At these times, you may feel like a single parent. It can be lonely and overwhelming to support both your partner and children.

Recognizing that being a parent may give your partner a great deal of meaning and purpose, you may consider encouraging rituals that they can do with your children. For example, they may go on walks or prepare Sunday brunch with the kids. Although encouraging such structured parenting activities is not your responsibility, both your partner and children may appreciate it.

Thinking about parenting with your partner, consider the following emotions and situations. Write in your experiences and feelings if you wish:

Frustration: *I feel angry when my partner* _____

_____

_____

Proud: *I feel proud of my partner when they* _____

_____

_____

Sadness or disappointment: *I feel sad when* _____

_____

_____

Resentment: *I resent* _____

_____

_____

Exhausted or overwhelmed: *When my partner is struggling emotionally, I sometimes feel*

_____

_____

Grateful: *I so appreciate when my partner* _____

_____

_____

Embarrassed: *Our kids are so humiliated when* _____

_____

_____

Afraid: *I don't know how to protect our kids when my partner* _____

_____

_____

Connected: *I feel close to my partner when* _____

_____

_____

Describe other emotions you feel in parenting with your partner: _____

_____

_____

> "I feel furious because my partner is checked out of our kids' lives—it's like he doesn't care."
>
> —A DAD

> "When our family goes out to dinner and my husband yells at the server for a small error in the bill, my kids and I want to disappear—it's so embarrassing."
>
> —A MOM

Common Impacts of Parental Mental Illness on Children

Kids whose parents have a mental illness experience a wide range of feelings. Just like the adults in the family, children and teens may feel confused, scared, sad, hurt, lonely, ashamed, worried, and angry. The unpredictability of their parent's behavior can be especially stressful, never knowing how their parent will act from one day to the next . . . or even one hour to the next. For example, sometimes the parent may spend days on end in bed, and the kids have no rules and free run of the house. Then, at other times, the parent is overprotective and won't let them go to their friends' homes. These changes in boundaries, expectations, and routines can be confusing and frustrating.

Has your partner's mental illness affected your children? If so, how? _____

_____

_____

What do you notice in your children when your partner is going through a difficult time?

_____

_____

_____

Along with having a wide range of feelings, kids respond in a variety of ways. Do you recognize your children in any of the following feelings and behaviors?

Struggling with strong feelings and questions

- Blame themselves: *What did I do to cause my mom's illness?*

- Feel hurt and confused: *Why won't Dad come to my tennis matches?*

- Be especially clingy: *If I keep trying to be good, maybe Mom will spend more time with me. I'm scared when she's not there for me.*

- "Act out" to get attention: *Because everyone seems so focused on Dad, maybe this will get their attention!*

- Worry: *Am I going to be like Mom someday?*

Trying to make family life more peaceful (be a "little adult")

- Walk on eggshells: *If I can be perfect and never make any mistakes, maybe Mom will stop getting so mad. I don't want to stress her out so she gets sick and has to go to the hospital again.*

- Try to fix their parent: *If I can just get my dad to take his pills regularly, I know he'd feel so much better. He's just a different person when he's on his meds. I help fill his pill organizer every week.*

- Take on adult responsibilities: *If only my little brother would stop being such a brat and quit annoying Mom! I try to keep him busy and quiet at home, but sometimes he has tantrums that upset her.*

Trying to separate themselves from the family

- Distance from the family: *Life at home is just out of control. I'd rather be anywhere than at home, so I spend most of my time at friends' houses.*

- Act as if they don't care: *I've given up—it's just too much. I don't give a darn if Dad gets help or not. There's really nothing I can do anyway.*

- Avoid having friends to the house: *What if Mom is drunk and drills my girlfriend with a million questions? It's so embarrassing!*

Are there other things you notice in your children's behavior? If so, describe here:

_____

_____

_____

Regardless of how your kids respond, they're doing the best they can in a tough situation. As a parent, taking the time to think through what's driving their behavior can help you respond with love and patience (even when their actions are upsetting). Remembering that your children are trying to cope with their strong emotions can help you to be understanding.

In sum, these challenges that you and your children may be experiencing are common and difficult. Prior to exploring eight strategies for supporting your children, let's take a look at how one family navigates maternal bipolar disorder.

The Hernandez Family

Consider the Hernandez family, including Anita, Manuel, and their daughter, Sofia:

Anita and Manuel met in New York City; she was performing in off-Broadway shows and he was in pharmacy school. They quickly fell in love, got married, and were excited to start a family.

Shortly after their daughter, Sofia, was born, Anita started having intense mood swings. She'd had some mild depression in the past, but this was entirely different. Some weeks, she'd stay in bed and cry much of the day; other times, she felt on top of the world, had tremendous energy, and made plans for amazing international family vacations. At first, she thought it was just post-partum moodiness, but the ups and downs didn't level out. Anita felt panicky when Manuel returned to work and wasn't sure she could handle Sofia on her own. Anita's favorite aunt had bipolar disorder, so the symptoms were familiar. Anita wondered if she might be developing the illness as well.

Manuel was scared and didn't know what to do. He'd never seen Anita like this, and worried about her ability to take care of Sofia. In addition to being exhausted and sleep deprived himself, he felt helpless to support his wife and baby.

Over the next few months, Manuel repeatedly encouraged Anita to see a psychiatrist, and she eventually agreed. The doctor gave her a diagnosis of bipolar disorder and suggested therapy and medicine. Although it took some time to find the right medication and dose, Anita felt more stable and more confident as a parent and partner. Manuel found support for himself in a NAMI class in his community. Talking to other family members helped him feel less alone and gave him hope.

For the first several years of Sofia's life, Anita had a long period of stability. She took her medicine regularly and learned skills in therapy to manage her mood swings. Although she definitely still had ups and downs, she and Manuel worked together to manage her illness. Manuel was relieved at how well Anita was doing, but always worried if her symptoms might return.

When Sofia turned six, Anita enrolled her in dance class. Sofia was excited when her mom became an assistant teacher. The first few months were awesome, and all of Sofia's friends loved her mom's energy and pizzazz! Sofia loved sharing dance with her mom and was so proud to have her as her teacher.

Shortly after Thanksgiving, Anita's mom died. Everything changed. The grief was intense, and she missed her mom terribly. Anita stopped taking her medicine and her mood swings returned. She withdrew physically and emotionally from Manuel. She insisted that she was taking her medicine, but he suspected otherwise—her sleep was irregular, she was pretty irritable, and she spent a lot of money purchasing frivolous items online.

At dance class, Anita started acting strangely. She disrespected the head instructor, talked too much, and became paranoid, thinking the other parents were talking about her. Sofia was scared and confused; this was not her mom! What happened? She'd never seen her mom like this before. Anita's behavior became so disruptive that the studio owner asked her to take a break from teaching. Sofia was embarrassed and didn't know what to say to her friends. At home, Sofia became clingy and didn't want to leave her mom's side. When Anita was crabby and withdrawn, Sofia felt lonely and confused. Sofia tried to cheer her mom up by drawing pictures, dancing for her, and giving extra hugs.

Before continuing with the Hernandez family story, let's consider specific ways parents can help their children.

Eight Ways to Support Your Kids and Help Them Cope

Figuring out how care for your partner, your kids, and yourself can be a lot to juggle, especially during rocky times. The good news is that kids are pretty resilient! The majority of children raised in families managing a mental illness do well. Research has found that resilient children tend to have strong social support, a sense of purpose, hope and optimism, active coping skills, a sense of belonging, good problem-solving skills, and the ability to regulate their emotions.[49] So, although having a parent with a mental illness can be a bumpy road, most children cope effectively.

However, we know that these youth are at higher risk for developing emotional problems themselves.[50] It's impossible to predict if any particular child will develop a mental illness because so many different factors come into play. Importantly, parents can take specific steps to help their kids, including teaching them how to understand and cope with feelings, recognizing early signs of more serious problems, and seeking treatment early. All of these steps can help children's long-term well-being.

Although an in-depth exploration of how to support children is beyond the scope of this book, we offer eight suggestions to help you as parents and to foster resilience in your kids.

1. **Take care of yourself.** The single best thing you can do as a parent is to take care of your own well-being. Being good to yourself helps you be present for your kids.

You are being a good parent when you are intentional about self-care. Not only are you improving yourself, but you are also being a good role model for your child. So, instead of feeling guilty for doing that yoga class after work, remember that committing this time for yourself is actually good for everyone!

2. **Spend time alone with your child regularly.** It can be helpful to schedule one on one time with your child on a regular basis. Your child can look forward to that quality time together. Although you may occasionally have serious conversations, dedicating this time to playing, having fun, and hanging out can strengthen your relationship. Of course, what you do together and the frequency of the shared time depend on their developmental level. (Some teenagers are most ready to talk at midnight!) You know your child and can suggest activities they will enjoy doing with you.

3. **Talk openly about the mental illness and offer information in bite-size chunks, using language your kids can understand.** Children are perceptive. Although they may not fully understand what they see and feel, they usually sense when someone is struggling. As children fear what they don't understand and often blame themselves, it's important for them to know what is going on. We believe it's important to be open and honest, using developmentally appropriate language. By naming and openly talking about the situation, you also have the opportunity to discuss how it's impacting them.

   Because these conversations can be awkward, you may want to ask for help from a professional, a family member, or a friend. Resources listed at the end of this chapter can help you with these discussions.

4. **Listen and encourage your kids to share their feelings and questions.** When you name the mental illness as the elephant in the living room, you open the door for children to share their feelings and ask questions. Although you may plan topics to address in specific conversations, your child may also raise the subject at random times, perhaps on the way to school or at bedtime. Be open to ongoing dialogue, and let them know you want to hear what they're thinking and feeling. The questions kids have and their reactions to mental illness change over time, so your explanations need to shift accordingly.

   As a parent, you may not know all the answers or what to say, and that's OK! You may consult with a professional or family member to think through how to respond. As children discuss and begin to understand their parent's illness, they may develop greater compassion and empathy for others, and may begin to appreciate that life can be uncertain at times.

5. **Offer reassurance.** In addition to being honest about the fact that your family is dealing with some challenges, it's important to offer reassurance. Although you decide what is appropriate for your unique situation, some helpful messages include

   - *You're not alone. Over 1 in 20 American adults has a mental illness like your mom or dad. Many families are affected.*

   - *You didn't cause your parent's illness, and it's not your fault.*

   - *We see you. We realize this situation affects you. We want to support you.*

6. **Create a support team for your children, possibly including their own therapist.** Your partner's mental illness can consume a lot of time and energy, which can result in your having less to give to your kids. Encourage your children to spend time with other kids and to explore their interests outside the home.

   You may also be intentional about creating a support team which may include their own individual therapist. Many other people can also help your children, such as family members, friends, faith leaders/elders, and community members such as coaches, teachers, and neighbors. These adults might create a regular ritual with your child (such as shooting hoops or getting ice cream together) or they may make themselves available when times are especially rough.

   Are there adults in your kids' lives who are especially supportive? If so, who?

   _____
   _____
   _____

   If not, who in your support network might be able to be there for your kids? Might you consider reaching out and asking them to be part of your team? _____

   _____
   _____
   _____

7. **When a crisis arises, ask for help.**

   What's helpful for you and your children when things are especially rough at home?

   _____
   _____
   _____

Remember, you don't have to go through hard times alone. Asking for help takes courage. People often want to support you but just don't know how. Be specific about what they can do to be helpful, such as picking up groceries, dropping the kids off at school, or spending time with your loved one so you can have some time alone.

8. **Empower your kids and instill hope.** It's important to approach conversations in an honest yet positive manner. Instill confidence in your children that they can manage this difficult situation and have coping tools for the tough times. As a parent, you know that sticking to daily schedules and routines can build resilience, but take breaks and be flexible when needed. Help your children focus on what they have control over.

Children can be comforted by optimistic messages such as

- *We have doctors, counselors, relatives and friends who are helping us during this difficult time.*

- *Mental illness is treatable. There are many medications and therapies that can help your parent to feel better. Although we don't have a cure right now, scientists and doctors are developing new treatments all the time.*

- *We've been through hard times as a family before—we can handle this!*

- *Although you can't cure your parent, there are ways you can help and support them. Your parent loves it when you* _____ (*fill in the blank with small things your child can do, such as give hugs, pick up their room, or send a loving text message*).

Now let's check in on the Hernandez family and see how they work together to support Sofia:

Anita, Manuel, and her health care team work hard to help Anita after her mom's death. She re-starts her medicine and joins a peer support group through the Depression and Bipolar Support Alliance (DBSA). Anita and Manuel begin couples therapy to learn to communicate better and work together to manage her illness. The therapist also suggests ways to talk with Sofia about bipolar disorder.

Anita carves out special time to be alone with Sofia after school. They play games and watch videos of famous dancers. Sofia knows she can count on this time with her mom, and sometimes they have heart-to-heart talks about Anita's well-being. Anita explains that four or five other kids in Sofia's class at school probably have a family member with a mental illness, so Sofia is definitely not alone.

Manuel also makes it a priority to have regular Daddy and daughter time; they have fun taking their dog on a walk and getting ice cream together. He notices that Sofia sometimes asks questions about her mom's health. In the back of his mind, Manuel worries that Sofia might develop bipolar disorder someday given the strong family history. He's aware of early warning signs and has a plan to quickly connect with her pediatrician if he notices any concerning behavior.

Anita and Manuel tell Sofia that there are many medicines to help people with a mental illness and that Anita has a strong team of helpers. Anita talks with Sofia's teacher and school counselor about her bipolar disorder and makes sure Sofia knows they are available if she wants to talk to someone at school. Sofia also knows she can always talk to her aunt or uncle; she loves visiting them and playing with their kitty.

Resources for Your Family and Children

As noted above, you may choose to seek professional help for your children as they deal with their parent's mental illness, perhaps including therapy:

- **Individual therapy** can give your child a chance to talk honestly about their feelings and receive support from an objective professional. Your child can learn how to identify and cope with emotions, and the therapist can monitor your child for behaviors that may be red flags for more serious problems. In general, the sooner potential problems can be identified and treated, the better.

- **Family therapy** can assist everyone in talking openly about their feelings and how they can work together.

In addition, several resources have been developed specifically for children. As you, your partner, and your children navigate this journey together, you may wish to consider the following books and organizations.

- **Interactive books for youth**
  - *I'm not alone: A teen's guide to living with a parent who has a mental illness or history of trauma.* 2nd edition. (2025). M. D. Sherman & D. M. Sherman. Seeds of Hope Books.
  - *Wishing wellness: A workbook for children of parents with mental illness.* (2006). L.A. Clarke. Magination Press.

- **Organizations** (websites include videos, blogs, family care plans, etc.)
  - Children of Parents with a Mental Illness (COPMI) (www.copmi.net.au)—based in Australia
  - Our Time: Helping young people affected by parental mental illness (www.ourtime.org.uk)—based in the United Kingdom
  - Lapproche, University of Quebec (www.lapproche.uqo.ca)—based in Canada

Part IV

MANAGING COMMON CHALLENGES

Chapter 13

WHEN YOUR LOVED ONE DOESN'T ACKNOWLEDGE THE ILLNESS OR DECLINES HELP

IN THIS CHAPTER, YOU WILL

✓ Learn what can make it hard for your loved one to acknowledge and accept their illness

✓ Consider barriers to seeking professional help

✓ Reflect on reasons people discontinue mental health medications

✓ Consider tips for talking with your loved one about accessing and sticking with care

✓ Reflect on your experience when your loved one declines professional help

People you love can make choices about their health that disappoint you. They just don't do what you think they *should do*. When that happens, you may feel frustrated, confused, and powerless. You may worry . . . a lot. You may try to motivate them to do what you think is best, such as dropping subtle hints, being encouraging, nagging, offering resources, and even getting very direct and confrontational.

Consider these situations.

- Your grandpa won't go to physical therapy after surgery.
  - *I'm worried he won't heal after having his hip replaced. Why won't he go to PT and do the exercises? What if he falls? I've even offered to take him to appointments, but he won't accept my help.*

- Your husband doesn't believe his high blood pressure could lead to problems.
  - *I'm so frustrated—I just don't get it! Although his blood pressure is high, he doesn't think it's any big deal and won't take the medicine the doctor prescribed. I've suggested we consider cooking low-sodium meals, but he is just not interested . . .*

Similar situations can occur when a loved one has a mental illness.

- Your husband tells the psychiatrist that everything is "fine." He doesn't share that he spends most of his time in his pajamas, dozing on the couch, downing energy drinks, and playing games on his phone.
  - *I'm really frustrated that he doesn't tell his doctor how bad his depression is . . . no one can help him until he shares what's actually going on . . .*

- Your daughter stopped taking her antidepressant and has started drinking again
  - *I'm just beside myself . . . she was doing so well when she was taking her meds! Ultimately, these are her decisions, but it's hard seeing her dark moods return . . .*

Are there things your loved one does (or does not do) regarding their mental health that concern you? If so, describe the situation and how you feel:

- My _____
  - I feel _____
    _____
    _____

- My _____
  - I feel _____
    _____
    _____

Acknowledging Mental Illness

Experiencing symptoms of mental illness, especially for the first time, can be scary. It's common to wonder: *What's going on? What caused this? Will this ever go away? What does this mean for my future? Am I going to be like my father who struggled with depression his entire life?* So many questions and feelings can emerge, including anger, confusion, shock, and sadness.

Additionally, as we discussed in chapter 4, people may experience shame and embarrassment about their mental health problems. Not wanting to consider the possibility of having a mental illness, people sometimes develop various explanations for their symptoms such as

- *It's just a phase.*

- *It's a midlife crisis.*

- *It's due to all the stress I'm under at work.*

- *I'm not depressed . . . I'm not sitting around crying all day! I'm just ticked off a lot and am not getting along well with my wife.*

- *This is normal for me; I've felt this way my whole life. This is just who I am.*

- *These problems are just because I drink too much; I can quit any time I want.*

Acknowledging mental health problems can be difficult and is usually not a one-time event. It takes courage to be honest with oneself and others.

A Note about Anosognosia ("uh no sog NOH zee uh")

While stigma, shame, and embarrassment can significantly impact the experience of mental illness and readiness to get help, there's a less well-known factor that is crucial to understand: some people do not believe they have an illness. Anosognosia is defined as **limited or no awareness or understanding of one's illness.**[51] This symptom is experienced by some people living with schizophrenia and bipolar disorder, and it is a common reason people are not interested in treatment or stop taking their medications. The level of insight can fluctuate over time. Anosognosia may be caused by damage to the part of the brain that is associated with self-reflection. Precise rates of this condition are not known, as findings vary considerably across studies. Estimates of prevalence are 30–58% among people living with schizophrenia and 20–40% for people who have bipolar disorder.[52]

Anosognosia can be confusing for family members and friends who feel frustrated and assume their loved one is just "in denial"—when, in fact, the symptom can be part of the illness. If your loved one has anosognosia, you may find the book *I Am Not Sick, I Don't Need Help! How to Help Someone Accept Treatment* by Dr. Xavier Amador[53] to be helpful. It describes the LEAP communication skills (Listen, Empathize, Agree, and Partner) which may be useful in encouraging a loved one to consider treatment. Information and videos describing this approach are available here: www.leapinstitute.org.

> "When my daughter was first sick, there was nothing her doctor or I could say to help her understand she was ill."
>
> —A DAD

Barriers to Seeking Professional Help

After someone has acknowledged that they are struggling and has realized they are not able to manage their problems on their own comes the next step—asking for help. This takes strength and courage. People may weigh the pros and cons of reaching out for professional help for months or years. When hurting emotionally, the pros may seem pretty weak, and the cons list may get long quickly.

Sadly, only about two-thirds of American adults managing a serious mental illness receive mental health services in a given year, meaning over eight million people with these conditions go without professional help.[54] Some people who don't get help become involved in the legal system and spend time in jail or prison—clearly not a comfortable environment for someone dealing with a mental illness. Unfortunately, the criminal justice system has become the largest provider of mental health services in the country.[55]

The sheer number and complexity of barriers to seeking professional help contribute to these stark statistics. Barriers may be logistical issues, fears, and beliefs. Starting and staying in treatment take time, energy, money, motivation, and some degree of hope.

Consider this list of common barriers and check those that you sense your loved one experiences (or has experienced in the past).

If your loved one has sought out care, they may have overcome many of these obstacles. Reaching out for help can takes humility and courage.

Barriers

Logistics

- I don't know what I need or where to get it.
- No mental health providers have any openings right now.
- I can't afford the therapy, doctor appointments, or medications.
- I can't find a therapist who speaks my language or understands my culture and values.
- I don't have transportation to get to appointments.
- I don't have anyone to watch my kids when I go to therapy.
- I work all day and can't get away for appointments.
- I don't have insurance, or my insurance won't cover it.

Fears

- I'm nervous telling a total stranger all of my problems; I'm a private person.
- If I start talking about my life, I'll cry and won't be able to control myself; I'm too ashamed.
- People in my culture don't go to therapy; asking for help will bring shame to my family.
- What if someone finds out that I'm going to therapy? In our family we don't talk about private matters with others.
- I don't want to be "locked up" (admitted to a psychiatric unit).
- I'm afraid I will be discriminated against or used in the name of "treatment" or "science."
- I worry about the implications of a mental health diagnosis being on my health record or insurance file. Might it hurt my career?

Beliefs

- Therapy is for "crazy people"—I'm not crazy!
- My parents say mental illness is a test from God; I just need to pray harder and talk to our church elders.
- Nothing will help. I've done therapy before and it didn't help. It's a waste of time and money. Why try?
- It would take too much energy; I can hardly get out of bed much less consider counseling.
- I should be able to handle this on my own.
- My situation isn't that bad—other people have it much worse and they need therapy more than I do.
- There's nothing wrong with me.

Reasons People Discontinue Mental Health Medications

In addition to these general barriers to seeking professional help, it's important to consider issues specific to psychiatric medications. The concerns listed here can prevent people from starting medications and can also lead people to stop taking them, which can worsen symptoms and may lead to a crisis.

Here are some common concerns people have about mental health medications:

- *I don't want to be put on a "mind-altering drug."*

- *What if I get hooked/addicted to the medicine?*

- *I just can't remember to take them. I forget to order refills.*

- *The side effects are miserable.*

- *The pills change me; I want my personality back.*

- *My insurance doesn't cover the medicine my doctor recommends.*

- *I like the energy I have when I'm manic—the pills make me tired, boring, and dull.*

- *I think these pills are bad for my physical health—I've gained so much weight, and I worry how they're affecting me.*

- *I don't think the medicine is doing anything.*

- *Taking the pills means I'm different from other people—it's like a daily reminder.*

- *I can't afford the medications.*

- *I don't have a mental illness (anosognosia).*

- *I feel better now so don't need to take them anymore.*

- *The pills I get on the street work better than the medications my doctor prescribes.*

Helping Your Loved One Access and Stick with Care

Chapter 7 described many suggestions for how to navigate the complex health care system. In this section, we offer tips on helping your loved one deal with emotional barriers to starting and sticking with treatment.

Four Tips on Talking with Your Loved One about Accessing Mental Health Care

1. **Listen.** Sometimes it's hard to know how your loved one feels about mental health treatment. Ask and be open to hearing their honest reactions—what they fear, dread, find helpful, consider a waste of time, and so forth. Try to set aside your opinions and agenda, listen with a nonjudgmental manner, and work to understand their perspective.

2. **Use their words rather than focusing on labels or diagnoses.** Some people strongly object to diagnostic labels such as *depression* or *schizophrenia* and names of symptoms such as *delusions* or *paranoia*. The dislike of such terms can be driven by stigma, shame, worries about their implications, and the lack of awareness of their illness (anosognosia). Genuine frustration among family members and friends is very understandable when a loved one objects to what seems like obvious symptoms. However, attempts to persuade them can damage your relationship and may actually further deter them from seeking care.

    We encourage you to give up this fight. It's just not important.

    Rather, listen for what is upsetting your loved one. For example, maybe they will acknowledge feeling stressed out or having a hard time sleeping. Use their words to show that you're listening and that you care. You can build upon this shared understanding to strengthen trust. Instill hope by noting how treatment could help with their stress and sleep. Increasing the likelihood that they will consider seeking help is far more important than accepting a label.

3. **Explore the WHY: How could treatment help your loved one move toward their goals?** Using your loved one's words, discuss why they might want to participate in treatment or take medications. How are their symptoms holding them back? How could better management or elimination of the symptoms enable them to work toward their goals? (Remember the tips on helping your loved one make progress toward their goals from chapter 6.).

It's also helpful to talk with your loved one about their values and purpose in life. For example, if your mom's depression is interfering with her ability to enjoy time with her grandchildren, talking about why she wants to gain better control of her sadness might help. Since being a loving and involved grandma is one of her most prized roles, exploring that value and the benefits of treatment can be motivating.

Because committing to treatment takes an investment of time, energy, and money, it's useful to focus on the "why"—why should your loved one do all this? How could it help? How might their relationships and quality of life be better if their symptoms were less intense or bothersome?

4. **Recognize the positive steps your loved one makes, and offer practical help.** Genuinely commend your loved one for their courage in seeking help, and be available to problem-solve if issues arise with treatment. Here are some specific messages that may be helpful:

- *I'm proud of you for scheduling that appointment with the therapist. It takes a lot of courage to ask for help.*
- *I know that taking the bus can be a hassle and Uber gets expensive; I'd be happy to drive you to the appointment.*
- *I use a pill organizer for my medicines and fill it every Sunday afternoon. You're so good at organizing things. I wonder if that might be helpful for you in remembering to take your meds.*

When Your Loved One Discontinues (or Wants to Discontinue) Care

Many people move in and out of treatment over time. Sometimes people participate in therapy or take medication for a while and then decide to take a break. Although it may be upsetting to see them discontinue care, especially if it leads to a relapse or crisis, this cycle is actually quite common.

Consider these scenarios of how your loved one might feel about their care and ways in which you could respond:

"No one is listening to me or asking what I want—they just throw pills at me."

➜ **Encourage your loved one to advocate for themselves.**
Dr. Patricia Deegan, a clinical psychologist who lives with schizophrenia, emphasizes the importance of people having a *voice* and a *choice* regarding their medications. Consistent with the recovery principles discussed in chapter 6, encourage your loved one to

talk with their provider about what they want the medication to do, such as to help them sleep better or relax.

Dr. Deegan encourages people to create power statements to convey their wishes. For example, your loved one could tell their provider: "I want you to help me find a medication that will help me _____ so that I can _____."[56]

If you wish to learn more about Dr. Deegan and her recovery academy, see her website which includes e-learning courses, videos, and recovery-focused resources (www.commongroundprogram.com).

Beyond just medications, all treatment decisions should be made as a team, grounded in ongoing discussion between your loved one and their provider.

"My provider just doesn't 'get' me."

→ **Express your concerns and consider switching to another provider.**
Dr. Deegan's perspective of "voice" and "choice" applies to all aspects of mental health treatment, not just medications. For example, emphasize that your loved one has a choice in their therapist and prescriber. If they don't feel listened to, understood, respected, or helped by their current health care team, encourage them to verbalize those feelings. If matters don't improve, it's definitely appropriate to explore other options. Chapter 7 has a list of online directories and resources to help locate treatment providers in your area.

"No one looks like me or understands my background."

→ **Explore culturally relevant services.**
Mental health services should be delivered in a culturally responsive manner, so people of all backgrounds and identities are seen, understood, and supported. Sadly, finding providers that are culturally competent for your loved one may be challenging. Be persistent in finding quality services that fit their needs. Chapter 7 also offers tips for finding culturally informed services and providers.

"Nothing is helping—it's taking forever!"

→ **Be patient.**
Getting an accurate diagnosis and finding a treatment plan that works can be a time-consuming process. Unlike with many physical health problems where tests and lab work can often yield a clear assessment, mental health concerns can be more subjective. It may take several appointments for the mental health professional to determine the appropriate diagnosis. Also, because people respond to medications differently, the

prescriber may try a few options to discover what is most effective with the fewest side effects. In addition, some medications take several weeks to reach full effectiveness, and waiting can be frustrating for everyone involved.

Your Experience When Your Loved One Declines Professional Help

Watching your loved one go through the ups and downs of a mental illness can be difficult, and dealing with their decision not to engage in treatment can be especially painful. Even though you may understand many of the barriers discussed in this chapter and feel empathy for their situation, it's common to have a lot of feelings about their choices.

How do you feel when your loved one chooses not to get help? Circle the emotion(s) you experience:

Angry	Confused	Impatient
Scared	Resigned	Frustrated
Understanding	Exhausted	Discouraged
Powerless	Hopeless	Other: _____

> "I felt devastated and frantic when my wife quit therapy and stopped taking her meds. I begged, cried, yelled, and pleaded with her, but nothing worked. I respect that it's her decision, but I worry she's going to spiral to a really dark place again—which is so painful for all of us . . ."
>
> —A HUSBAND

As Exhausting as It Can Be, Try to Hold onto Hope and Encourage Your Loved One to Seek Help

Shining a light on painful topics takes courage, but avoiding them doesn't work in the long run. People with a mental illness can become defensive, angry, embarrassed, ashamed, and more distant when someone asks about their illness and getting help. Let's face it, listening openly and responding in a nonjudgmental manner to constructive feedback can be challenging for everyone; taking this information to heart may be even harder when experiencing mental health concerns.

Even though your intent in these conversations is to be helpful, you may be accused of nagging and meddling in their private affairs. If your loved one responds in anger or spirals into a darker place, you may question yourself and wonder if you should have raised the topic at all. The situation may feel even worse than before you talked about it. Despite your best efforts at being supportive, having your loved one ignore, deny, or angrily push back on your suggestions can be painful.

Even if a conversation doesn't go as you had anticipated, try to feel good about opening up the dialogue, assuring yourself that you were coming from a place of love and support. If you feel hurt after a difficult conversation, reach out for support and use the coping tools discussed in chapter 2 and appendix B (Activities that Can Lift your Spirit).

Respect Your Loved One's Choices and Release Efforts to Control

Ultimately, your loved one's journey with their illness is unique and personal. How they choose to manage the illness is their decision. As much as you might like to, you cannot decide for them or hit the "fast forward" button. Just as you cannot yell at a flower to grow faster, you cannot hurry people along in their mental health journey; people grow at their own pace. You can only control yourself and your choices.

Respecting your loved one's decisions and grappling with powerlessness may be a challenging part of your journey. We encourage you to try to find the balance between being a supportive advocate and taking care of yourself. As explored in Chapter 10, sometimes it's a daily recommitment to releasing your efforts to control, focusing on being in the present, and showing up in love for your loved one and yourself.

Chapter 14

ADDICTIVE BEHAVIORS INCLUDING ALCOHOL AND DRUG USE

PAIN HURTS . . . BE IT THE PHYSICAL DISCOMFORT of a migraine headaches or the emotional pain of depression. Interestingly, research has found that the same parts of the brain are activated when we have physical discomfort as when we have painful emotional experiences (such as grief at a loved one's death, bullying, or social rejection).[57] Taking a couple of aspirins to get rid of a bad headache seems logical and common sense; we want to stop the physical pain quickly. Is the strong desire to eliminate emotional pain any different?

We often try to stop the pain by doing things that helped in the past. After a rough day at work, going shopping or having a couple beers may be relaxing and distracting. Shopping and drinking alcohol can be fun, and there's usually nothing harmful about enjoying them in moderation. However, difficulties can emerge when people need to do more and more of the same behavior to get the relief or good feelings they crave. Further, as will be explored in this chapter, excessive drinking, misuse of prescription medications, use of marijuana, and use of illegal drugs (such as cocaine, heroin, and methamphetamines) can create additional problems for people with a mental illness.

What are Addictive Behaviors?

People sometimes turn to addictive behavior to escape painful life circumstances. The initial drive to self-medicate can spiral into an addiction. Common features of addiction include

- Continuing the behavior despite harmful consequences, such as problems with physical health, mental health, work performance, or relationships

- Needing to do more and more of the behavior to get the same effect

- Feeling unable to control the behavior—wanting to stop but being unable to do so

- Having cravings and urges to engage in the behavior

- Experiencing withdrawal when stopping the behavior

Although we often think of addictions in relation to alcohol, prescription medication, and illegal drugs, people can develop problems with many different issues such as gambling, nicotine, pornography, sex, video games, work, and exercise.

We believe that human beings are doing the best they can at any given time. The addictive behavior may appear confusing and even self-destructive to an outsider, but it may be the best way the person knows how to manage their emotional pain at the time.

Addictive Behavior and Mental Illness

Addictive behavior can serve many different functions for people with a mental illness or a history of trauma. Escaping emotional pain, quieting upsetting symptoms, and perhaps even feeling numb may be very appealing. Seen in this way, the behaviors make a lot of sense. For example:

- *Smoking calms my nerves.*

- *Having a few drinks before bed helps me fall asleep faster.*

- *Buying random stuff online gives me a little joy when I feel super depressed . . . but sometimes I just can't stop . . .*

- *Marijuana seems like the only thing that stops the voices.*

- *Playing video games for hours is a great escape from life.*

- *Working long hours at two jobs keeps my mind busy and distracts me from thinking about my traumatic experience.*

- *Using cocaine gives me energy—it's just so good to feel happy again.*

Now, take a moment to consider these questions:

Does your loved one engage in any addictive behavior(s)? If so, what? _____

_____

_____

What is your perspective on how the addictive behavior helps your loved one (what function does it serve)? _____

_____

_____

What are the negative impacts of addictive behavior on your loved one? _____

_____

_____

Alcohol and Drug Use

Although people living with a mental illness may engage in a variety of addictive behaviors, problems with alcohol and drugs are especially common. Therefore, the rest of this chapter focuses on misuse of substances, including alcohol, prescription medication, and drugs.

National surveys report that approximately 1 in 10 American adults have had one or more substance use disorders (addiction to alcohol or drugs) in the preceding year.[58] The

COVID pandemic has been associated with significant increases in both the frequency of heavy drinking[59] and rates of death due to drug overdoses.[60] Substance-use disorders are real brain disorders and can be chronic for some people.

Importantly, among people with a mental illness, use of marijuana and illegal drugs can cause problems, *even if the person has not developed an addiction to the substance.* Many drugs can heighten symptoms, reduce medication effectiveness, and decrease overall motivation.

Impacts of Substance Misuse on Your Loved One

As shown in the figure below, misuse of substances can impact all aspects of life, including mental health, work and school performance, relationships, parenting abilities, physical health, and spiritual well-being.

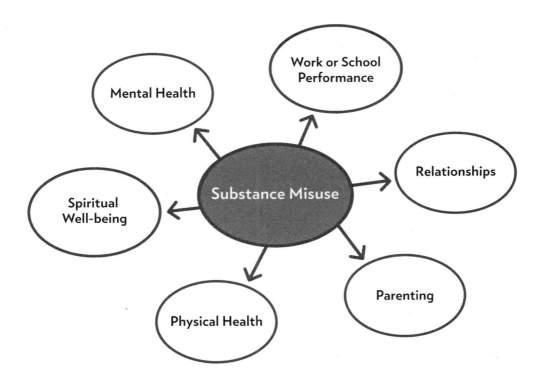

If your loved one misuses alcohol or drugs, consider how their well-being has been affected in these six areas. If you wish, take a moment to write about what you have observed: _____

Impacts of Your Loved One's Misuse of Substances on You

Now that we have considered how your loved one's substance use has affected their life, let's focus on your experience.

Has your loved one's misuse of alcohol or drugs affected you? If so, how?

_____

_____

_____

What has been most challenging for you? _____

_____

_____

How has it impacted your relationship with your loved one? _____

_____

_____

    You may experience many of the emotions discussed in chapter 1 when your loved one is drinking too much, using marijuana or illegal drugs, or using prescription medications inappropriately. Consider the following common feelings among family members and friends.

Complete the sentences that speak to you:

Worry or fear: *I'm afraid that* _____

_____

_____

Sadness: *It hurts me that* _____

_____

_____

Anger: *I'm angry that* _____

_____

_____

Guilt: *If only I* _____

_____

_____

Powerlessness: *The situation feels so out of my control—it's like there's nothing I can do. If only*

_____

_____

_____

Confusion: *I just don't understand why* _____

_____

_____

Hope: *I'm so glad my loved one* _____ *and hope that* _____

_____

_____

Other emotions you experience: _____

_____

_____

Co-existence of Substance Use Disorders and Mental Illness ("Co-occurring Disorders")

There's a great deal of overlap between mental illness and substance use disorders. In fact, over 17 million American adults experienced both a substance-use disorder and a mental illness in 2020.[61] These two kinds of illnesses are closely intertwined. The mental illness or substance-use disorder doesn't necessarily cause the other, and sometimes it's hard to know which develops first.

Although alcohol and drugs can provide short-term relief from emotional pain, they can negatively impact people with a mental illness in many ways, such as

- Cause or worsen mental health symptoms, including
  - Mood: anxiety, depression, apathy, low motivation, mood swings
  - Thinking: paranoia, hallucinations, delusions
  - Behavior: angry outbursts, irritability, social withdrawal, restlessness
  - Feelings about oneself: shame, guilt, low self-confidence

- Impair judgment which can result in poor decisions

- Increase the risk of violence (to self and others)

- Increase the chance of discontinuing mental health treatment

- Reduce the effectiveness of mental health medications

- Make accurately diagnosing the mental health problems more challenging

Let's consider the Meyer family as they manage a mental illness and alcohol misuse.

Wyatt and Dawn's dairy farm in rural Wisconsin has been in the family for four generations. Wyatt has always enjoyed farming, but the long hours, unpredictable weather, and decreased revenue have been extremely stressful; in fact, the farm hasn't seen a profit in three years. Wyatt has become deeply depressed and doesn't have the energy to manage the many farming responsibilities. He has gone through some down periods in the past, but nothing quite like this. He has also started drinking more and hides the empty bottles in the barn.

Wyatt's wife, Dawn, has seen the changes in him and is really worried. She knows he's stressed about the rising costs of feed and supplies. Although she knows he drinks to escape, the more he drinks, the more depressed he becomes. With finances being so tight, Dawn is also angry that he spends so much money on alcohol.

Dawn would love Wyatt to talk to a professional—but he is such a proud, private man; he doesn't like to admit any weaknesses or ever ask for help. And, even if he were open to therapy, the nearest clinic is 75 miles away. Dawn feels powerless as to how she can help. She's considering talking to a friend from church whose husband recently had some similar problems, but she is fiercely protective of Wyatt and worries that rumors might fly if others learn what is going on.

Responding to Your Loved One's Upsetting Behavior

People who misuse substances can make choices that have ripple effects on others. They may minimize or deny their use, lie, act in secretive ways, and blame others. As their use progresses, efforts to obtain and use more of the drug can become all-consuming, and their behavior may be inconsistent with their core values. For example, a trustworthy son who has never stolen anything might take money from your wallet to buy drugs. His need for the substance and his fear of withdrawal can drive extreme behaviors.

Seeing your loved one act in these ways can be painful; they may not seem at all like the person you know! Your ability to trust them may be damaged, and you may feel scared, hurt, and angry. Your loved one may ask you to help them, such as purchasing alcohol, bailing them out of tough situations, or giving them money.

Knowing how to respond and best support your loved one can be very hard. Part of you wants to help them and understands the difficult situation they are in; because you love them, you may feel desperate to do anything to relieve their pain. However, you also know that enabling them and fixing their recurring crises aren't beneficial in the long run.

Ultimately, it's up to your loved one to decide if and when they change their use of substances. Nagging, crying, threatening, and persuading generally don't work. Remember a key message from Al-Anon: *I did not cause it, I can't control it, and I can't cure it.*

Supporting someone who misuses substances is beyond the scope of this book. However, we offer the following pointers and encourage you to check the resources described in appendix F.

- Give specific positive reinforcement when your loved one is not using. Share how you enjoy being together when they are sober, and suggest activities you know they enjoy.

- When your loved one is drinking or using, leave the situation and do something else. For example, you could say *"I'm going to take the kids to the park because I don't enjoy spending time with you when you are drinking."*

- Use good communication skills such as being specific, brief, optimistic, and understanding (check out chapter 9 for more tips on communicating effectively).

- Setting limits with your loved one can be very hard but is often a loving and appropriate choice. For example, you may set a limit that they cannot bring drugs into your house. You may find the guidance on limit setting in chapter 10 to be useful.

- Make your own well-being a priority! Remember the coping tools and wellness suggestions described in chapter 2 and appendix B (Activities to Lift your Spirit), as well as the family support opportunities listed in appendix F.

Accessing Treatment in a Crisis

People in the throes of addiction usually cannot just "stop" or "quit," and abrupt cessation may be dangerous. Due to the medical risks associated with withdrawal from many substances, seeing a health care provider can be important. Depending on the situation, inpatient or closely monitored outpatient detoxification ("detox") may be appropriate.

If you are unsure how to access care at a time of crisis, options include

- Calling or texting **988**, the Suicide and Crisis Lifeline, to talk to a trained crisis counselor

- Calling 911 if anyone is in immediate danger

- Going to a local emergency room

- Checking the Substance Abuse and Mental Health Administration (SAMHSA)'s website (www.findtreatment.gov) or calling their 24/7 anonymous hotline (1-800-662-HELP)

Note: If your loved one is misusing opioids, you may wish to have Narcan nasal spray on hand in case of an overdose. It is a medication that can reverse the effects of an opioid overdose, and is intended to be used by family members or friends without medical training. You can purchase Narcan at the pharmacy without a prescription.

Supports for You and Your Loved One

Historically, mental illness and substance misuse were treated separately. For example, people were told to "get sober" or "go to rehab" and then their depression would be treated afterwards. However, current treatment approaches address the issues simultaneously (see appendix E for a list of many effective models).

As explored in this chapter, you may be greatly impacted by your loved one's behavior. You may take comfort in knowing that many services are now available to support the entire family (see appendix F). You can learn helpful skills such as how to set limits, improve communication, reinforce non-drinking and non-using behavior, be supportive during crises, and avoid enabling.

COMMUNITY REINFORCEMENT AND FAMILY TRAINING (CRAFT)

In particular, we encourage you to consider the Community Reinforcement and Family Training (CRAFT) model, an approach in which family members and friends learn skills to modify how they interact with their loved one who is misusing substances. Importantly, this model is focused on supporting the family member or friend, not the person with the substance-use problem. Key components of this approach include communication skills, rewarding non-using behavior, negative consequences for using behavior, goal setting for one's own well-being, and looking for windows of opportunity to talk with the loved one about engaging in treatment.

Research on CRAFT with both alcohol and drug misuse has found that 40–60% of family members and friends report that their loved one engaged in treatment within a year; they report improvement in their own well-being as well.[62-63] To learn more about this treatment, including books, a provider directory of trained therapists, and details about online groups, see their website: Helping Families Help (www.helpingfamilieshelp.com).

A NOTE ABOUT SUPPORT GROUPS

Many people find peer support groups to be a helpful part of recovery from substance use problems. Numerous groups are available for both the person who is drinking/using (e.g., Alcoholic Anonymous or AA, SMART Recovery) and the people who love them (e.g., Al-Anon, Helping Families Heal, Alateen). Many groups are offered both in-person and virtually. Here are a few pointers about groups:

- Most people feel anxious when going to a new group meeting—but then find comfort in connecting with other people facing similar challenges. Groups can be a place to both give and receive information and support. It's very possible that something you share in a group might be just what someone else needs to hear.

- As with any resource, the first group or program you try may not be a good fit. Every 12-step meeting has its own culture, norms, and vibe. Look around until you find somewhere that you feel you belong and are understood.

- Some groups convey the viewpoint that mental health medications are not appropriate for people in recovery. If this sentiment is expressed, we encourage you to consider finding another group as that stance is not universally held and is not consistent with the science of recovery.

Let's return to the Meyer family and see how Dawn found some support for herself:

> Dawn's friend from church told her about an online Al-Anon meeting that she found helpful, so Dawn checked it out. She was nervous and didn't really know what to expect. She just listened during the first few meetings and found herself relating to the stories she heard. It was great to be reminded that she is not alone, and she learned helpful tips for how to take care of herself and support Wyatt with his

depression and drinking. After a while, she began sharing a bit of her own experiences and feelings. Joining the virtual meeting was so simple—no worries about childcare, Wisconsin winter roads, or gas prices—and it only took an hour out of her busy day.

A NOTE ABOUT INTERVENTIONS

Interventions are an approach some family members and friends use to try to get people with substance use problems into treatment. Concerned relatives and friends prepare and stage a meeting in which they share how the addiction has impacted them and urge the loved one to start treatment. Sometimes families hire a professional interventionist to facilitate the process. Due to the confrontational approach and risk of negative outcomes, however, we urge caution. Rather, we encourage you to draw upon your personal and professional support networks and the skills provided in this book when talking with your loved one about treatment.

Remember: Neither you nor your loved one have to walk this journey alone. See appendices E and F to learn about many different treatment and support programs.

Chapter 15

POSSIBLE IMPACTS OF TRAUMA (INCLUDING POST-TRAUMATIC STRESS DISORDER)

LIFE EVENTS SUCH AS DIVORCE or being fired from a job can be very upsetting, and people sometimes describe them as "traumatic." However, in the mental health field, the term "trauma" is more narrowly defined. It refers to exposure to threatened or actual death, serious injury, or sexual violence. The person could have experienced the event personally, watched it happen to someone else, or learned that a close family member or friend experienced it.[64]

Traumatic events can include many different experiences, including but not limited to military combat, car accidents, terrorism, natural disasters (earthquake, flood, hurricane), sexual assault, violent crime, domestic violence, physical or sexual abuse, and human trafficking. Trauma can also be experienced by first responders, such as firefighters and police, who regularly encounter dangerous situations.

Over 80% of American adults experience at least one traumatic event at some point in their life.[65] Fortunately, most people don't develop long-term difficulties. However, people with a mental illness experience trauma and develop lasting problems at much higher rates than the general population.[66]

If your loved one has experienced a traumatic event(s), name it here if you wish:

_____

_____

IN THIS CHAPTER, YOU WILL

✓ Consider common reactions to trauma

✓ Learn about post-traumatic stress disorder (PTSD), including
   ○ Symptoms
   ○ Impacts on you, your loved one, and your relationship
   ○ Tools for supporting your loved one and caring for yourself

✓ Read about treatment options for PTSD as well as
   ○ Post-traumatic growth
   ○ How to support your loved one in treatment

Common Reactions to Trauma

Experiencing, witnessing, or learning about a traumatic event can be very frightening. Almost everyone is shaken at first. Distressing thoughts, images, dreams, feelings, and sensations are very common in the first few days and weeks.

To repeat: _most people don't develop long-term problems_. They can usually draw upon their coping tools, support network, inner strength, and sometimes spiritual or religious beliefs to get through the difficult time and return to daily routines. However, some people experience lasting challenges that affect their overall well-being, relationships, worldview, sense of meaning or purpose in life, spiritual or religious beliefs, academic or work functioning, and life satisfaction.

Although it's impossible to predict who will develop mental health difficulties after a traumatic event, some risk factors include a very intense or long-lasting trauma, being physically injured, a history of previous trauma, and pre-existing mental illness such as depression or anxiety. In addition, people who tend to isolate from others or avoid feared situations may be at greater risk of developing emotional problems after a trauma.

On the other hand, protective factors can buffer people from long-term problems. These can include seeking support from family or friends, using positive coping strategies, and, if possible, finding some meaning in the trauma (the concept of post-traumatic growth is described in the last section of this chapter).

As shown in this picture, trauma can result in a variety of mental health issues; people often experience several of these problems at the same time. In addition, trauma can make pre-existing conditions worse.

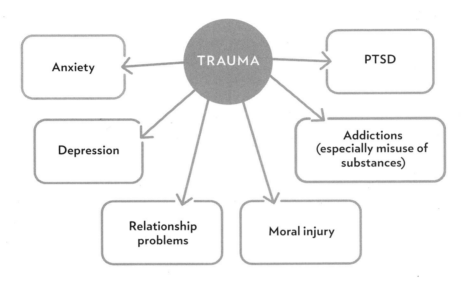

More specifically, reactions to trauma can involve

- **Anxiety:** Muscle tension, panic attacks, restlessness, discomfort in crowds or around people, worry such as wondering when something bad might happen again

- **Depression:** Sadness, guilt, sleep problems, loss of interest in enjoyable activities, problems concentrating

- **Relationship problems:** Difficulties with communication, trust, and physical or emotional intimacy; increased conflict

- **Moral injury:** Guilt, shame, spiritual distress and/or anger related to having done or witnessed something that violated one's core values, morals, and beliefs

- **Addictions:** Misuse of alcohol or drugs, gambling, pornography, etc. (see chapter 14 for more on addictive behavior)

- PTSD

Because PTSD can have considerable impacts on relationships—and often co-exists with other mental illnesses—the rest of this chapter focuses on this condition.

Let's meet the Robinsons, firefighter Darnell and his wife, Kiara. We follow their story throughout this chapter.

> Darnell is a 60-year-old firefighter who has served his community fire department for 30 years. In addition to working fires, he loves going to schools to teach about safety and fire prevention. Although Darnell has worked many fire calls, one in particular has haunted him for several years—the house was destroyed and a young girl died.
>
> Darnell has been married to Kiara for 35 years; they have two grown daughters and two adorable granddaughters. Kiara has always supported Darnell in his firefighting, and she is proud of his service to their community. She worries about him when he gets a call but takes comfort in knowing his unit is well trained. Although Darnell rarely talks about what happens, she knows that one particularly bad fire continues to trouble him.

Post-traumatic Stress Disorder

PTSD is a mental illness that can develop after experiencing a traumatic event. About 1 in 15 Americans (6%) develop PTSD at some point in their lives.[67]

People with a mental illness experience more traumatic events than the general population; in addition, they are at higher risk of developing PTSD after experiencing trauma.[68] The reasons for these increased risks are not known but may relate to being more vulnerable and having fewer effective coping strategies. In addition, people who have experienced trauma or PTSD can have a more difficult course of mental illness—more intense symptoms and a higher risk of misusing alcohol and drugs.[66]

PTSD symptoms can be organized in the following four categories. It can be helpful to use the acronym RAIN (created by Dr. A.L. "Dutch" Doerman, Colonel in United States Air Force, Retired):

Re-experiencing the trauma

Avoiding thoughts, feelings, and reminders of the trauma

Increased reactivity and irritability

Negative feelings and thoughts

For each of these categories, we will

- Describe common symptoms

- Invite you to reflect on your loved one's experience of those symptoms, as well as the impacts on you and your relationship

- Explore Darnell's experience

- Consider Kiara's experience

- Provide tips for supporting your loved one and taking care of yourself

Re-experiencing the Trauma

Trauma survivors can re-experience the event in many ways such as upsetting memories, nightmares, and flashbacks (feeling like the event is happening again). Sometimes the trigger is clear such as an anniversary or reminder of the trauma; other times, however, it may seem like the thoughts and feelings come out of the blue.

Do you know if and how your loved one re-experiences their trauma? If so, describe:

_____

_____

_____

What are those times like for you? Describe your experience, as well as what helps you cope.

_____

_____

_____

Darnell's Experience: Memories of that horrific night come to Darnell a couple of times a week, especially when his unit is called to the same neighborhood as the fatal fire. Seeing children that resemble the girl who died also spikes his anxiety; his blood pressure goes up, and he feels tense and clammy. Darnell has nightmares of seeing the child's face; he sometimes thrashes around in bed and breaks out in a cold sweat. When he wakes up, he feels exhausted and upset.

Kiara's Experience: Darnell's nightmares are scary and troubling for Kiara. She hears him yell in his sleep as he cries out to the other firefighters and the girl's parents. It seems so real—like he's re-living the fire. She wants to hold and comfort him but doesn't know what to do.

TIPS FOR YOU

- You may or may not know when your loved one is re-experiencing their trauma. You might notice them appearing distracted, "zoned out," agitated, or pre-occupied. Try to respect *if* and *how much* they want to talk with you.

- Realize how upsetting these nightmares, flashbacks, and memories may be for your loved one. For a minute, think about re-living the very worst thing that has ever happened to you—over and over. Vivid images, feelings, thoughts, and sounds come to you out of nowhere. No way around it—these can be terrifying.

- The following suggestions may be helpful when they experience flashbacks and nightmares:
  - If your loved one agrees, you might develop a game plan together for how you can be supportive when they have distressing memories.
  - You may use "grounding" techniques to help them re-connect with the present. Using a calm, quiet tone of voice, ask them the date, location, and your name. You may talk about things in your surroundings to help connect with the here and now. You may also encourage them to connect with their senses by talking about what they see, hear, feel, and smell in their present environment.
  - In general, it's best to avoid touching your loved one during a nightmare or flashback. If they are threatening or engaging in any violence, protect yourself, your children, and your pets—you may decide to leave the room or house.
  - Realize your loved one may feel embarrassed and ashamed after the flashback or nightmare. Showing understanding, grace, and kindness can be good ways to be supportive. For example, Kiara might say: *"You're a good man, Darnell, and I love you. You've saved many lives as a firefighter, and the community holds you in high regard. We will get through this together."*

Avoiding Thoughts, Feelings, and Reminders of the Trauma

Trauma survivors often want to avoid things that remind them of the event, which can include both external reminders (people, places, and activities) and internal reminders (thoughts and feelings).

Are you aware of places, people, or activities that your loved one avoids? If so, describe:

_____

_____

_____

What do you notice about how their avoidance affects their quality of life? _____

_____

_____

_____

How does their avoidance affect you? _____

_____

_____

Darnell's Experience: Kiara and Darnell have always been active in their church. Since the fire, Darnell often finds an excuse to avoid going to Sunday morning service, saying he has a headache or just doesn't feel like it. They used to enjoy a nightly ritual of walking their dogs around the block, but he's no longer interested in that either. He also stopped teaching fire safety at the local elementary schools, an activity he used to love. All he really wants to do is hibernate in his office and play video games.

Kiara's Experience: Kiara is confused and frustrated. She wonders if Darnell is angry with her. She questions what she did wrong. She feels lonely, not knowing why he won't go to church or on walks. She goes to service by herself, but it's awkward when the minister asks about Darnell—she doesn't know what to say.

TIPS FOR YOU

- Don't let your world become smaller! Respect if your loved one does not want to engage with other people and activities but stay connected with your support network and things that give your life meaning. It's understandable that you may feel guilty at times, but remember that it's not helping you, your loved one, or your relationship for you to become isolated.

- Respect that your loved one may not want to talk openly or often about their traumatic event. They may feel more comfortable talking to other trauma survivors than to you. Avoid asking questions regarding the details of their trauma; it's important to follow their lead regarding if and how much they want to share.

- "Exposure" is a common part of therapy for PTSD that involves helping people "face their fears" and confront scary situations. Although doing so can be frightening, it helps people re-train their brains to understand that the situations are safe and that avoidance is no longer necessary. You can support your loved one to re-engage with previously feared experiences by providing encouragement and positive reinforcement. Details about therapy options are provided at the end of this chapter and in appendix F.

Increased Reactivity and Irritability

Experiencing a traumatic event can challenge your view of the world as a safe, predictable place. For example, although walking around the mall may have always felt comfortable, an assault can shatter that sense of safety. Consequently, trauma survivors often feel tense and revved up. Relaxing and letting one's guard down can feel risky and vulnerable.

People who have experienced trauma may struggle to sleep and have a hard time concentrating. They can be especially irritable or crabby, and may even become aggressive at times. Trauma survivors may also startle easily and feel the need to be hypervigilant or acutely aware of what's going on around them. These symptoms can make being in groups or crowds uncomfortable, so people may avoid social settings such as restaurants, grocery stores, or sporting events.

Do you notice your loved one being especially tense? Or having a short fuse? Or having strong reactions that seem out of proportion to the situation? If so, describe:

_____

_____

_____

What is that like for you? _____

_____

_____

Darnell's Experience: Since the fire, Darnell has felt pretty stressed out and edgy. His migraines returned, and his primary care doctor cautioned that his blood pressure had gone up. Darnell used to love long weekends at the lake with Kiara and the kids and grandkids, with fun nights of board games, s'mores by the fire, and pontoon rides. Now, he spends hours preparing the firepit area to make sure it's safe and won't let anyone help. He can only tolerate games for a short time before he gets angry and stops playing. He also gets irate when his grandchildren come up from behind and surprise him. To escape the chaos of the cabin, he often takes long walks in the woods by himself.

Kiara's Experience: Kiara feels like she is walking on eggshells—she never knows when Darnell will fly off the handle. She tries to keep her granddaughters quiet so they won't upset Grandpa. Her stomach is often in knots, unsure of what might set him off. She misses the way the family used to have such fun together at the lake. Kiara hardly recognizes him—what happened to her laid back, fun-loving husband who looked forward all year to the family weekends at the cabin?

TIPS FOR YOU

- Find relaxing activities that you and your loved one can do together, perhaps being in nature, playing cards, or going on a leisurely drive. Spending quiet time together can be calming and good for your relationship.

- Avoid surprising your loved one, such as coming up behind them without their knowing.

- Consider taking two cars to events so your loved one can leave early if they wish and you can stay and enjoy yourself. If your loved one chooses not to attend, go on your own. Don't let your loved one's PTSD make your life small.

- When you go to social events, discuss in advance what might help your loved one feel comfortable (such as sitting near the back of a theater or restaurant, so their back can be to the wall and so they can see the exits).

- Set limits if your loved one is especially irritable or angry. Having PTSD does not make it OK for them to treat you disrespectfully. If you and your loved one get into an argument that escalates, remember the Time Out process described in chapter 10.

- Violence of any kind is NEVER OK (please see the resources in chapter 16 and the Resource List if you ever feel in danger). PTSD is not an excuse to treat anyone in an abusive manner.

Negative Feelings and Thoughts

Trauma survivors can develop an overall negative perspective that can affect many aspects of their lives—feeling negatively about themselves, other people, the future, and the broader world. Given this negative lens, they may experience depression, lose interest in activities they used to enjoy, and become isolated.

Do you notice that your loved one tends to be negative—such as anticipating the worst, being down a lot, and feeling hopeless? Perhaps they have discontinued hobbies or activities they used to enjoy? If so, describe: _____

_____

_____

_____

What is your experience of being around that negativity? Are you able to prevent that energy from consuming you? If so, how do you keep your spirits up? _____

_____

_____

_____

Have you discovered any ways of gently challenging your loved one's negative perspective? Perhaps by using humor, distraction, reminders of your blessings, or messages of hope? If so, describe: _____

_____

_____

_____

Trauma survivors can also struggle to experience and express positive emotions, such as love, joy, or happiness. At other times, they may feel numb or nothing at all. Because feelings are what connect us to other people, this lack of emotion can lead to distant relationships without much vulnerability and intimacy. Strong feelings of guilt and self-blame, which can be out of proportion to the situation, are also common among trauma survivors. Some people who have experienced life-threatening situations develop survivor guilt, wondering why they lived through the trauma when others did not.

Do you sense that your loved one struggles to share their feelings with you? If so, what is that like for you? _____

_____

_____

_____

Have you discovered activities or situations in which your loved one is more open or comfortable in sharing their thoughts or feelings? If so, describe: _____

_____

_____

_____

> ## "It is a lonely feeling when someone you care about becomes a stranger."
>
> **LEMONY SNICKET**[69]

Darnell's Experience: Darnell questions himself every day as to what he could have done differently to have saved that child in the fire. Even though he knows from his training and 30 years of experience that he did everything he could, he lives with a lot of guilt. He seems to have lost his purpose, energy, and spunk. Nothing is fun anymore, not even playing with the grandkids. He used to be excited for them to come over, but now he retreats to the den and watches TV when they visit. He knows he is checked out as a husband and has no interest in physical intimacy. He wonders why Kiara stays around.

Kiara's Experience: Kiara feels like she has lost her partner and best friend. The energy around the house has changed, and it's frankly depressing to be around Darnell. They used to have a fun banter as they lovingly teased each other, but now he is sullen and withdrawn; they live more like roommates than anything else. He's there—but not there. Kiara feels abandoned, lonely, and sad.

TIPS FOR YOU

- As hard as it may be, recognize that your loved one's withdrawal is most likely due to their trauma and PTSD and not a reflection of you or your relationship.
- Spending a lot of time around someone who is especially negative can bring your own spirits down. Be sure to commit energy and time to your own well-being.
- When your loved one is unable to be supportive of you, seek validation, friendship, and encouragement elsewhere. You need and deserve to be cared for! You can give and receive love in many ways—children, grandchildren, siblings, parents, pets, friends, volunteering, or spiritual activities.
- Let your loved one know that you miss them and want to reconnect. Depending on your relationship, you may consider couples therapy with a provider who has expertise in trauma.

Treatment Options

Several effective psychotherapy treatments and medications can help trauma survivors cope with these RAIN symptoms and move forward with their lives. Many therapies involve the survivor directly confronting the upsetting memories, usually through talking or writing about the event(s).

Because one of the core symptoms of PTSD is avoidance, the idea of facing the trauma head on can be daunting. However, repeatedly doing so with the guidance and support of a therapist can lessen the impact of the event and help people manage their symptoms. Of course, people never forget the traumatic event, but therapy can help so that the trauma does not define, control, or constrict their lives.

Appendix F (Family Education Programs and Support Groups) describes a wide array of resources, including specific options for PTSD. In addition, the website of the National

Center for PTSD (www.ptsd.va.gov) has extensive, research-based information for families and friends.

Further, there are some couples therapy approaches that aim to both decrease PTSD symptoms and strengthen the relationship. Two excellent models with growing research support include Cognitive-Behavioral Conjoint Therapy for Post-traumatic Stress Disorder (CBCT for PTSD) developed by Drs. Candice Monson and Stephanie Fredman, and Structured Approach Therapy (SAT) created by Drs. Fred Sautter and Shirley Glynn.

Post-traumatic Growth

Sometimes trauma survivors come to recognize and appreciate ways in which they have grown in the process of recovery. Scientists have termed this post-traumatic growth.[70] Although not universal and in no way denying the very real distress associated with the experience, post-traumatic growth may involve an increased appreciation for life and second chances. People may feel proud of their strength in coping, and be grateful for the people who have supported them.

Have you noticed any positive changes in your loved one? If so, what have you seen?

_____

_____

_____

Have you noticed any improvements in your relationship? If so, describe: _____

_____

_____

_____

Have you shared these observations with your loved one? If so, how did it go? _____

_____

_____

Supporting Your Loved One in Treatment

Therapy for PTSD can be challenging, and it may be hard to know how to support your loved one. Remember they are facing their past in order to create a more positive future, a process that takes courage and strength. Letting them know that you respect and admire their hard work can go a long way.

If your loved one is tempted to discontinue therapy, acknowledge that their work in counseling sounds very difficult and encourage them to discuss these feelings with their therapist. Sometimes symptoms can be more intense in the early phases of therapy—it can feel like things are getting worse rather than better—when, in fact, that is a common part of the healing process. Overall, follow your loved one's lead on if and how much they want to share about their experience of therapy.

Let's return to Darnell and Kiara and their experience of seeking professional help.

Over time, Darnell's symptoms were getting worse. He felt like a stranger in his own house. He talked to a good friend from the fire station and shared what was going on. His friend said that he had gone through a lot of similar stuff a few years back, and he found counseling to be very helpful. He warned Darnell that therapy was hard, but it was totally worth it.

Darnell got the name of his friend's therapist and scheduled an appointment. The therapist told him about a treatment called Prolonged Exposure, which is a kind of cognitive behavioral therapy. He would learn how to approach his memories, feelings, and thoughts about the fire rather than avoid them. Darnell was nervous and knew it would be difficult, but he wanted to get his life back, let go of some guilt, and be part of his family again. Kiara was proud of him for being willing to try therapy and hopeful it would help.

Darnell completed the Prolonged Exposure treatment and found it very helpful. Although it was definitely challenging, it wasn't as difficult as he feared, and his therapist was very supportive. He no longer needed to avoid so many situations, was less haunted by his memories and nightmares, and was finally able to relax and enjoy his family more.

Darnell and Kiara wanted to work on their relationship, so they went to couples therapy with a marriage and family therapist who has expertise in trauma. Through these sessions, they gained tools that strengthened their relationship, including how to better communicate, solve problems, and deal with issues of trust and intimacy, For example:

- Kiara told Darnell how she missed enjoying church services and walks together. He shared that seeing the kids at church and the park is uncomfortable, as they remind him of the girl who died in the fire. Kiara was grateful for his honesty. They decided to try going to church together online for a while; they also took a different route for their walks that does not pass by the park.

- They both committed to noticing what their partner does that they appreciate. Being intentional about "looking for the good" helped shift the focus from the negativity to a more positive outlook.

- Over time, Darnell has grown more comfortable with the energy at the cabin when the grandkids visit. With therapy, he has become less triggered and startled by noises and is able to enjoy time with the family. Instead of escaping by himself to the woods, he now brings his grandkids along on walks and enjoys sharing the beauty of nature with them.

- Kiara just beams when she sees Darnell playing with the grandkids. She's so proud of him and the courage it took to work through his trauma. They still have tough days and know their relationship will continue to take work, but she's hopeful about their future together.

Chapter 16

MENTAL HEALTH CRISES

MENTAL ILLNESS OFTEN GOES IN CYCLES. People may feel well for many months or years; symptoms are lessened or managed, perhaps bolstered by peer support, therapy, supportive relationships, regular physical activity, medications, healthy eating, and/or enjoyment of meaningful activities. Then, a difficult phase comes along; sometimes the cause is clear such as the death of a loved one, divorce, job loss, increase in use of alcohol or drugs, stopping medications, or a traumatic event. However, at other times, it's hard to pinpoint an exact trigger. Your loved one may be consistently taking their medications and participating in treatment, but a crisis can still arise. This unpredictability can be really hard.

Although mental health crises can take many forms, they generally involve periods of feeling overwhelmed and struggling to cope effectively. The specific behaviors depend on the illness(es) and often pose some risk to oneself or others. For example, trauma survivors or those with post-traumatic stress disorder (PTSD) may become very tense or even aggressive during flashbacks or nightmares (see chapter 15 for tips on responding to these frightening experiences). Manic episodes among people with bipolar disorder can involve intense mood swings and extreme behaviors, such as spending sprees and reckless driving. Crises among people with schizophrenia can involve confusion and aggressive behavior, sometimes driven by auditory hallucinations (voices they hear that others do not).

IN THIS CHAPTER, YOU WILL

✓ Identify your loved one's warning signs of a potential crisis

✓ Consider who to contact in crisis situations

✓ Learn how to create a crisis plan

✓ Reflect on strategies for dealing with times when your loved one
  ○ Engages in self-harm or suicidal behavior
  ○ Threatens or engages in violent behavior
  ○ Is admitted to the hospital

✓ Explore how you can cope with especially challenging times

Warning Signs

It's helpful to understand and recognize warning signs that may foreshadow a crisis for your loved one. In reality, symptoms change over time, and having a few rough days usually doesn't result in a crisis. However, helping your loved one to manage stress well, be aware of their warning signs, and get help early can sometimes prevent a mental health emergency.

As part of your loved one's illness, they may not recognize certain behaviors in themselves. It's possible that you notice the changes before they do. When warning signs first start to emerge, encourage your loved one to use their coping tools and draw upon their support network.

What are the warning signs that your loved one may be really struggling? See chapter 2 for a list of symptoms and behaviors that may be red flags. _____

_____

_____

What do you sense is helpful for your loved one when they are going through a tough time? _____

_____

_____

In addition to you, who else can your loved one turn to for support? _____

_____

_____

If the warning signs don't improve or your loved one struggles to keep up with their routines, it's probably time to reach out to a professional for help. Of course, severe symptoms (such as suicidal comments or behavior, violence or threats thereof, difficulties with activities of daily living, or psychotic symptoms) warrant immediate attention.

Who Should You Contact?

Sometimes it's hard to know who to contact when you're concerned about your loved one, especially when emotions are high. Specific resources differ by community, and you may want to explore what is available in your area during a non-crisis time. However, the following guidelines apply more broadly:

- If *there is immediate danger* and you're concerned for the safety of your loved one or anyone else, go to the emergency room or call **911** immediately. Specifically say that this is a mental health emergency.

- If *there is no immediate danger*, **988** is the Suicide and Crisis Lifeline which connects callers with trained counselors. This Lifeline is available 24/7 and is for people in crisis AND those who care about them. Other options in non-emergent crises include alerting their psychiatrist or psychiatric nurse, therapist, caseworker, or other mental health professional.

Suicide and Crisis Lifeline: Call or text 988

- Many communities have **Crisis Intervention Teams** (**CIT**) composed of police officers and sometimes mental health professionals and peer support specialists who have special training in working with people experiencing a mental health crisis. When you call for assistance
  - Be clear that it's a mental health crisis
  - Describe specifically what your loved one is doing
  - Ask for a CIT officer

- When you reach out for help in an emergency, there is no guarantee that law enforcement or the crisis team will take your loved one to the hospital. The more specific information you can provide about your loved one's mental illness and recent behavior, the better. Even if your loved one is brought to a crisis center or hospital, there is also no guarantee they will be admitted. In many states, if your loved one is not deemed an "imminent danger" or is not voluntarily seeking help, there is little the police or health care team can do . . . which can be extremely upsetting for you. It can be helpful to learn about your state's civil commitment laws which can mandate treatment (see appendix E for more information).

Crisis Plans: Planning for Future Tough Times

Because crises can be stressful and frightening, you may wish to create a crisis plan together. Taking the time to prepare in advance can help make the situation more manageable. Identifying low-level warning signs is important; it's easier for you loved one to get back to baseline if they get help when symptoms are mild rather than waiting until the situation escalates.

Create this plan together during a calm time, when things are going well. Personalize it to your needs, including information that is most relevant for your loved one.

Crisis plans can include

- Regular wellness activities

- Coping tools

- Warning signs

- Support system—family, friends, peers, and professionals

- Plans for managing crises (doctors' and therapists' phone numbers, caregivers for kids, list of medications, etc.)

Reviewing and regularly updating this plan can ensure its usefulness over time. If appropriate, you may share it with others who are closely involved with your loved one. During a non-crisis time, talk with your loved one about signing a Release of Information form which enables open communication between you and the treatment team, both routinely and during emergencies.

As discussed in chapter 3, you may also encourage your loved one to create a psychiatric advance directive in which they can define their preferences for future mental health treatment and/or designate a representative to make decisions about their treatment if they are unable to do so. The National Resource Center on Psychiatric Advance Directives (www.nrc-pad.org) has up-to-date information by state on how to create these directives, and you may wish to engage a local attorney for assistance. You may find the free mobile app, My Mental Health Crisis Plan, to be helpful in creating and sharing such a document.

Consider the following crisis plan that Pedro and his partner, Emmanuel, created as they work together in managing Pedro's bipolar disorder. They save and regularly update the plan on an online shared account, making it readily available if a crisis arises.

Pedro's Crisis Plan

Wellness activities: Get 7–8 hours of sleep per night. Go on a 20-minute walk three days/week. Take my pills after breakfast. Meditate before bed.

Coping tools: Reach out to a friend from AA. Play with the kids. Talk to Emmanuel.

Warning signs: I know I'm starting to go downhill when my sleep gets messed up and I stay up for days on end . . . or when I start talking super-fast and cannot focus. When this happens, I need to ask for help because my medicine may need to be adjusted.

Support system:
- Family: Emmanuel (partner), Isabella (mom), Gabriela (sister)
- Friends: Julio (boss), Lisa (neighbor), Chaplain Damian (church)

Peer and professional support:
- Therapist: Dr. Torres at Care Counseling
- Peer support: Noah (peer support specialist)
- Psychiatrist/nurse/doctor: Dr. Luke at Care Counseling
- Primary care provider: Dr. Sanchez at the Allina clinic

Plans for managing crises (call or text 988 to talk to a trained crisis counselor, or call 911 if anyone is in immediate danger):
- **Hospital I would like to go to if needed:** United Hospital

- **I want Emmanuel to:** Remind me that going to the hospital really helped me last time—I felt so much better after my meds were changed. Tell my boss, my mom, and my therapist that I'm in the hospital.

- **I don't want Emmanuel to:** Get bossy and tell me what to do . . . or judge me. Don't tell my friends at church about my hospitalization.

- **Who can help with our kids:** My sister

- **My current medications** (name and dose): Lamotrigine 150 mg/day for bipolar disorder, Lisinopril 20 mg/day for high blood pressure

Having reviewed the importance of warning signs, who to contact in various emergency situations, and how to create a crisis plan, the rest of this chapter focuses on three common crises: self-harm and suicidal behavior, violent threats and behavior, and hospitalization. The chapter concludes with specific recommendations on how you can cope during these stressful situations.

Self-Harm and Suicidal Behavior

Suicide is the 12th twelfth leading cause of death in the United States.[71] People with a mental illness are at increased risk of engaging in self-harm behavior, attempting suicide, and dying by suicide.[72]

Self-harm behavior (also known as self-injury) involves deliberately hurting one's body. People who injure themselves are not always trying to end their lives. Rather, they may be trying to release strong feelings, punish themselves, or escape from emotional pain. Common types of self-injury include cutting, burning, or scratching oneself; punching or banging one's head; and pulling out one's hair. Often people feel ashamed and guilty after harming themselves, which can worsen the difficult emotions that initially triggered the self-injury behavior.

In contrast, suicidal behavior is usually motivated by a desire to die. People may experience deep depression, feel hopeless and alone, and sense that they are burdening others. Some people hear voices saying to harm or kill themselves.

Having someone you love talk about suicide or harming themselves can be terrifying. You may feel unsure of what to do, how to keep them safe, and where to get emergency care. It can be hard to know when to try to handle the situation on your own versus when to seek professional help.

Has your loved one talked about harming themselves or ending their lives? Has your loved one engaged in some kind of self-harm or suicidal behavior? _____

_____

_____

If so, describe what those experiences were like for you. What was the hardest part?

_____

_____

_____

How did you cope? _____

_____

_____

Although the complexities of dealing with a loved one's self-harm and suicidal behavior are beyond the scope of this book, we offer a few important suggestions:

- Asking about suicide does NOT plant the idea in someone's head. If you wonder if your loved one might be thinking about suicide, ask specifically: *"Are you thinking about killing yourself?"* Listen, show compassion, and connect with crisis resources if appropriate.

- Avoid debating the meaning of life or giving advice. Rather, let your loved one know that they matter to you. Offer hope. Don't promise to keep their suicidal thoughts a secret.

- You may pay attention for warning signs of suicide such as
    - Talking about wanting to die
    - Seeming especially hopeless, guilty, or agitated
    - Engaging in risky behavior
    - Talking about being a burden to others
    - Purchasing a gun or researching ways to die
    - Making or updating a will
    - Giving possessions away

Importantly, sometimes people act impulsively with little or no warning. Predicting if someone will actually harm themselves is very difficult, even for mental health professionals. Therefore, take all threats seriously and err on the side of caution in seeking professional help.

- If you are worried about your loved one, try to limit their access to potentially dangerous items such as guns, sharp objects, medications, alcohol, and drugs.

- Even if you suspect your loved one may be acting in a manipulative fashion, such as a "cry for help," step out of the conflict and focus on their safety. Sometimes people who don't necessarily intend to end their lives can seriously harm themselves.

- Encourage your loved one to seek help on a voluntary basis, and offer to drive or accompany them to the clinic or hospital. If you have determined they are in danger, however, do not leave them alone or let them drive themselves. If they are not willing to get help voluntarily, call 988 or 911 as described in the preceding section, "Who Should You Contact?"

- Realize that your loved one may be angry when you reach out and involve professionals. That's OK. It's better for them to be alive and upset with you than for you to have not taken action and live with guilt, wondering if you could have prevented their death. Remember: you're acting in love, you're taking their welfare seriously, and you're getting help from an objective professional who knows how to handle crises.

Supporting a loved one who harms themselves in any way can be highly stressful. You may question or blame yourself, be unsure how to help, and experience a wide range of emotions. The last section of this chapter offers tips for how to get through these especially challenging times.

An excellent resource aimed at supporting people affected by suicide is the American Foundation for Suicide Prevention (www.afsp.org). They conduct research, offer public education, and advocate to bring hope to people affected by suicide, and their website has many helpful resources.

Violent Threats and Behavior

Most people with a mental illness do not behave in a violent manner.[73] Many are generally fearful and avoid conflict or violence. However, some people act aggressively at times, and the behavior may be directed at family members and friends. This can include verbal attacks, threats, or physical violence.[74]

Risk factors for violent behavior among people with a mental illness include active substance misuse, past violent behavior, discontinuation of treatment or medications, impulsivity, and psychotic symptoms such as feeling persecuted or hearing voices directing them to harm someone.[75]

Knowing how to respond to a loved one's violent threats or behavior is also beyond the scope of this book. However, a few important points include

- Violence of any kind is **never** acceptable. You deserve to be safe.

- Mental illness is not an excuse or rationalization for abusive or aggressive behavior. Although your loved one may blame the illness for their behavior, such as "Well, I have PTSD . . . , " that does not make it OK.

- Violence can occur in many ways: physical violence (or threats), taking advantage of you financially, aggressive or inappropriate sexual behavior, and verbal or emotional abuse, which can include name-calling, criticism, humiliation, yelling or screaming, threats, ridicule, blaming, isolating you from friends or family, gaslighting, refusing to take responsibility for their behavior, and manipulating you.

- After the immediate crisis has passed, you may want to consider setting some firm limits or taking a break from the relationship. Although doing so can be difficult, it may be in everyone's best interest. You could also find an individual therapist to be invaluable in getting support and exploring your next steps.

- You may wish to create a safety plan, including somewhere you can go and someone you can contact 24/7. As it's hard to think clearly in the middle of a crisis, having a plan

If You Ever Feel Unsafe

If you are ever afraid, remove yourself, your children, and any pets from the situation, and call or text 988 (Suicide & Crisis Lifeline) or **911** if there's immediate danger. Rather than waiting to see if the situation will spiral out of control, leave at the earliest sign of potential violence.

Don't tell your loved one to leave—take the initiative and physically leave yourself. Avoid trying to reason with your loved one when they're upset. Attempting to calm them down when they are agitated usually does not work. Rather, give them space, leave the room or house, and seek support.

The **National Domestic Violence Hotline** has advocates available 24/7 to provide support and connect you with local resources. They can be reached via phone: 800-799-7233, text (text "start" to 88788), or chat via their website (www.thehotline.org). These programs can offer emotional support and strategies to protect you and your family.

in place can be useful. The following resources can guide you in creating a safety plan:
- The National Domestic Violence Hotline: 800-799-7233: www.thehotline.org
- National Coalition Against Domestic Violence: www.ncadv.org/personalized-safety-plan

Hospitalization

For some people managing serious mental illness, periodic hospitalizations can occur. Avoid framing your loved one's hospital stay as a failure. Recovery is not linear, and people benefit from different levels of care across time.

Being admitted to a psychiatric unit can be a culmination of several rough weeks or months. Sometimes people experience so much stress that life feels unmanageable. Stopping medication or using alcohol or illegal drugs that limit the medications' effectiveness can also result in an admission. In those situations, a brief hospitalization can be an excellent time to observe how a new medication (or dose) will work for your loved one. Suicidal thoughts or impulses may render the person unsafe and in need of the 24/7 observation and support provided by an inpatient unit. While admissions for mental health reasons are generally quite brief, they can allow for trials of new medications, more intensive counseling, and exploration of post-discharge treatment options.

Has your loved one been hospitalized for mental health reasons? If so, how did you feel during that time? _____

_____

_____

While your loved one is in the hospital, it can be helpful for YOU to

- Take the time they are in the hospital to re-charge, sleep, and rest.

- Try to let the health care team take responsibility for your loved one. Consider limiting phone and electronic communication and visits, especially in the first couple days of their stay at the hospital. Even if your loved one asks you to visit, it may be in everyone's best interest to give them space at first.

- Ask about visiting hours, as well as possible age restrictions on visitors; some sites do not allow young children on the unit. Talk to the social worker if you believe it would be helpful for your kids to visit, as exceptions may be possible.

- Communicate openly and regularly with the doctors, therapists, and social workers. Remember that you can give information at any time, and most health care providers value your input and questions.

- Ask about being part of family sessions and treatment team meetings. You may participate in discharge planning, including giving information about your loved one's past positive and negative experiences with different treatment approaches and advocating for what you think would be most helpful. Remember: you know your loved one far better than anyone else, and your voice is important.

Let's return to Pedro and Emmanuel and their experience of a hospitalization:

Pedro is admitted to the psychiatric unit once every couple of years to help stabilize and adjust his medication for bipolar disorder. The weeks leading up to the hospitalization are usually very stressful, so Emmanuel feels relieved when Pedro is admitted. He takes that time to catch up on sleep, go on long walks with the kids, and tinker on his old cars in his garage. Getting this extra rest helps Emmanuel to be supportive when Pedro comes home.

Coping during Challenging Times

Having explored the stressful experiences of a loved one's self-harm and suicidal behavior, violent threats and behavior, and hospital admissions, the rest of this chapter focuses specifically on your experience.

In addition to the general coping strategies discussed in chapter 2, the following suggestions may be useful for managing these particularly tough times.

Remember Everyone Is Affected— Give Yourself and Others Grace!

- Remember you're doing the best you can in a stressful situation.

- Although sticking to routines and schedules can be helpful, please give yourself some slack! Remember that you have a limited amount of time and energy, so some things will probably fall through the cracks. That's OK.

- Give others in the family extra grace as well. Remember that people respond differently to crises, and there's no "right way" to get through hard times.

- If children are involved, know they are also affected by what's going on, even if they don't fully understand or show it. Attempt to make extra time for them or engage others to offer a bit of extra support. Find ways to talk to your kids in developmentally appropriate ways about what is going on. Chapter 12 offers many tips on how to support children, as well as books for youth whose parent has a mental illness or PTSD.

Ask for Help and Watch Out for Red Flags in Yourself

- Talk to trusted friends or family members.

- Accept help. Allow others in your support network to assist you! People often want to help—you don't have to face difficult times alone. Be specific about how they can help you; let them know what you need.

- Explore opportunities to connect with others who love someone living with mental health problems. You may want to consider the National Alliance on Mental Illness or the Depression and Bipolar Support Alliance (more details in appendix F).

- Consider seeking professional help for yourself.

- Be aware of changes in your habits that may be red flags indicating that you are struggling. Monitor potentially risky behaviors involving alcohol, cigarettes, caffeine, drugs, gambling, shopping, or internet/social media/gaming activities. Most of these behaviors aren't problems in moderation. However, monitor if they're interfering with your daily responsibilities or if you're turning to them to escape.

Take Care of Your Spirit

- Remember to focus on what you have control over—and work to let go of what you don't (including your loved one's choices and behavior).

- Treat yourself to something special, perhaps a manicure, professional sporting event, massage, favorite meal, bubble bath, or night out with friends.

- Enjoy nature.

- Be physically active.

- Consider meditation or spiritual practices.

Be Open to the Possibility of New or More Intensive Treatment Options

As noted earlier, a crisis can be an opportunity to re-evaluate your loved one's treatment plan, possibly opening doors for new approaches, medications, and therapies. Appendices E and F list a wide array of treatment approaches and models, both for you and your loved one. Specific therapies can be helpful if your loved one routinely deals with issues of self-harm, difficulties managing strong emotions. or frequent hospitalizations:

> For your loved one: *Dialectical Behavioral Therapy (DBT)* is a structured, research-based psychotherapy that teaches skills for managing distress, improving interpersonal relationships, dealing with strong feelings, and being mindful in the present moment.[76] Many mental health clinics offer DBT programs, which usually involve a combination of individual and group therapy and support for managing crises.
>
> For you: The *Family Connections Program* is a free, evidence-based course for adults who love someone living with traits of borderline personality disorder (BPD) or emotion dysregulation. The person managing the illness does not participate in the program. In addition, a full diagnosis of BPD is not required. Courses are offered in-person or virtually and involve education, skills training, and support. More information is provided in appendix F.

You may also find the *Mental Health First Aid (MHFA)* one-day class to be helpful. Sponsored by the National Council for Mental Wellbeing, it educates and offers skills for recognizing and dealing with mental health and substance use crises. A schedule of courses can be found on their website (www.mentalhealthfirstaid.org).

WRAP-UP

WE HOPE THIS BOOK PROVIDED a safe place to reflect, learn, write . . . and perhaps cry . . . and perhaps hope. We trust that reading about others' experiences reminded you that you are not alone.

As the book comes to a close, you may wish to check in with yourself.

WHAT DID YOU LEARN

About yourself? _____

_____

_____

_____

About how to take care of yourself and keep your own well-being a priority? _____

_____

_____

_____

About how to support your loved one? _____

_____

_____

_____

Has the experience of supporting your loved one helped you grow as a person, or perhaps reminded you of your resilience? For example, Mitul Desai writes about his experience of supporting his brother who manages schizophrenia. He said that loving someone with a mental illness can provide "a unique opportunity to find deeper levels of resilience, empathy, and even gratitude—all superpowers for life." He added that his "family has endured a never-ending series of disappointments and all manner of emotional and physical strain—but we've also learned the value of persistence and emotional resilience."[77] Of note, Desai served as a Senior Advisor to Fountain House, a national mental health nonprofit organization dedicated to championing the dignity and rights of people living with a serious mental illness; it has over 200 social rehabilitation programs (clubhouses) across the country.

HAVE YOU EXPERIENCED GROWTH IN ANY OF THESE AREAS?

_____ Reminded you of your strengths

_____ Gave you opportunities to stretch yourself

_____ Challenged you to grow in patience, compassion, and hope
(even when it's hard)

_____ Helped you appreciate your support network

_____ Challenged or strengthened your religious or spiritual beliefs

_____ Led you to become involved in advocacy in some way

_____ Others? _____
_____
_____
_____

HOW WOULD YOU LIKE TO MOVE FORWARD?

To sustain your energy and well-being, it will be important for you to _____
_____
_____

You want to learn more about _____
_____
_____

You hope _____
_____
_____

Are there any action step(s) you are ready to take now? If so, describe here: _____

_____

_____

_____

What could get in the way? _____

_____

_____

_____

How might you overcome those obstacles? _____

_____

_____

_____

Who could help you? _____

_____

_____

_____

Although you have finished this book, your journey will continue. Perhaps you will come back and re-read your reflections or write more in the months and years ahead.

Please be gentle and compassionate with yourself, and remember to dedicate time and energy to your own well-being. Strength to you on your journey.

Michelle and De Anne

APPENDICES

Appendix A
FEELING WORDS

Appendix B
ACTIVITIES TO LIFT YOUR SPIRIT

Appendix C
SELF-ASSESSMENT OF OVERALL WELL-BEING

Appendix D
ADVOCATING TO FIGHT STIGMA AND DISCRIMINATION

Appendix E
MENTAL HEALTH PROFESSIONALS, SERVICES, AND SUPPORT GROUPS

Appendix F
FAMILY EDUCATION PROGRAMS AND SUPPORT GROUPS

Appendix A

FEELING WORDS

afraid	determined	frustrated
angry	devastated	furious
annoyed	disappointed	grateful·
anxious	discouraged	guilty
apprehensive	disgusted	happy
ashamed	disrespected	heartbroken
burned out	edgy	helpless
calm	embarrassed	hesitant
comforted	empathetic	hopeful
confident	empowered	hopeless
confused	exasperated	humiliated
content	excited	hurt
crabby	flustered	impatient
depressed	frantic	isolated
despair	frightened	jealous

joyful

lonely

loving

nervous

numb

offended

overwhelmed

panicky

paralyzed

peaceful

proud

rejected

relaxed

relieved

resentful

sad

self-conscious

shocked

stressed

surprised

tense

terrified

thrilled

unappreciated

weary

worried

worthless

ACTIVITIES TO LIFT YOUR SPIRIT

Go to a play or concert

Organize your drawers or cabinets

Do a crossword puzzle or word search

Volunteer at a local food bank
or pet shelter

Stretch or do yoga

Doodle or draw

Go to the gym

Have coffee with a friend

Meditate or pray

Join a local community choir or
theater group

Sew

Get a massage

Go for a walk, hike, or run

Get or give yourself a manicure

Play cards or board games

Try a new recipe

Play with your pet

Go to the park or library

Write a list of things that went well
in the past week

Get a car wash

Go golfing (or mini golfing)

Take a class

Contact a peer support counselor

Play frisbee golf

Wash your car

Watch a sporting event

Dance

Take a bubble bath

Go to a museum

Spend time in nature

Make a gift for someone

Make a video on your phone

Swim

Ride a bike

Go for a drive

Join a pick-up game at local park or gym

Listen to a podcast or audiobook

Make a list of things you're grateful for

Go shopping

Hang out with friends

Go on a picnic

Take a nap

Write a letter to someone who has made a positive impact on your life

Go bowling

Write or read poetry

Watch a funny video

Light candles

Buy fresh flowers

Donate old clothes or household items

Go to a movie

Visit a nursing home

Do woodworking

Join an advocacy effort

Listen to music

Repeat a loving kindness mantra ("May I be peaceful, safe, healthy")

Cook something special

Plant a garden

Call a crisis hotline

Play video games

Clean your house

Go fishing

Read a book, magazine, or blog

Do a Pay-It-Forward

Play an instrument

Rearrange the furniture in your house

Color in a coloring book

Fly a kite

Take care of your plants

Go out to dinner

Bake cookies

Write in a diary or journal

Appendix C

SELF-ASSESSMENT OF OVERALL WELL-BEING

WHEN SUPPORTING A LOVED ONE managing a mental illness, it's easy to become disconnected from yourself. So much of your time and energy are focused on them that you might not take the time to check in with your own well-being. Perhaps in neglecting yourself, you might miss signs that you are struggling as well.

This activity invites you to reflect upon your satisfaction with several parts of your life. First, rate your overall satisfaction with each domain. Then, rate each item on the 1–5 scale. If an area is not relevant, please skip it.

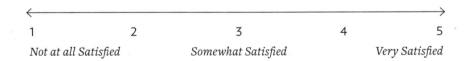

1	2	3	4	5
Not at all Satisfied		*Somewhat Satisfied*		*Very Satisfied*

Physical Well-being

Overall physical health

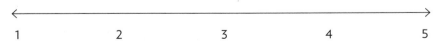

1	2	3	4	5

How satisfied are you with your ability to

_____ Sleep well and feel rested

_____ Make choices about your eating and diet that are healthy for your body

_____ Get regular physical activity

_____ Monitor or limit your use of caffeine and alcohol

_____ Keep up with regular doctor and dental appointments

Intellectual and Occupational Well-being

Overall intellectual and occupational health

$$\longleftarrow \hspace{8cm} \longrightarrow$$

| 1 | 2 | 3 | 4 | 5 |

How satisfied are you with your ability to

_____ Focus and concentrate

_____ Complete tasks and projects

_____ Solve problems as they arise

_____ Learn and be challenged intellectually

_____ Derive meaning and satisfaction from your work or volunteer activities

_____ Balance your work–life responsibilities with the time and energy you dedicate to supporting your loved one

Relationship Well-being

Overall relationship health

← ——————————————————————————————— →

1   2   3   4   5

How satisfied are you with your ability to

_____ Feel connected to family members

_____ Feel connected to friends, coworkers, neighbors, etc.

_____ Ask for help

_____ Be vulnerable and share your feelings

_____ Respect and value differences, approaching others with curiosity rather than judgment

_____ Be assertive and create boundaries when needed

_____ Laugh and play with others

Emotional and Mental Well-being

Overall emotional health

← ——————————————————————————————— →

1   2   3   4   5

How satisfied are you with your ability to

_____ Manage anger effectively

_____ Experience joy

_____ Cope with stress

_____ Have enough energy and motivation for your routines

_____ Participate in activities that give your life meaning and purpose

_____ Be kind to yourself when you're struggling

_____ Make time for yourself to recharge your own battery

_____ Maintain your own emotional stability when your loved one is struggling

Social Well-being

Overall social health

$\longleftrightarrow$

| 1 | 2 | 3 | 4 | 5 |

How satisfied are you with your ability to

_____ Participate in groups or social activities where you feel you belong

_____ Access safe parks and green spaces for recreation and connection

_____ Give back to your community via volunteering or advocacy activities

_____ Connect with other people who have a loved one living with a mental illness

Spiritual Well-being

Overall spiritual health

$\longleftrightarrow$

| 1 | 2 | 3 | 4 | 5 |

How satisfied are you with your ability to

_____ Feel a sense of meaning and purpose in your life

_____ Make time to reflect on your values—what's truly important to you

_____ Feel connected to something larger than yourself

_____ Draw upon the strength of your ancestors, family traditions, or spiritual beliefs

_____ Participate in spiritual or religious services, ceremonies, or other rituals

_____ Experience a sense of gratitude and awe

Financial Well-being

Overall financial health

←————————————————————————→
1   2   3   4   5

How satisfied are you with your ability to

_____ Live within your means

_____ Spend money in a way that aligns with your values and goals

_____ Know how to access community resources for financial assistance if needed

_____ Save for the future

_____ Manage stress surrounding financial challenges

_____ Have work that is meaningful

As you reflect on these types of well-being, you might choose to dedicate some time to a couple of areas that you rated as a 1 or 2. You could consider setting a goal to make some changes. You might decide to pursue your own therapy for support in strengthening your well-being.

When setting goals, it's helpful to

- Select a goal that is specific and challenging but not impossible
  - *I will walk for 15 minutes, three times a week.*

- Ask for support from someone who can hold you accountable
  - *I will ask my neighbor to walk with me on Mondays.*

- Anticipate barriers and consider ways to overcome them
  - *I will walk at the mall if it's raining.*

- Remember WHY you're setting this goal (How does this activity relate to what's important in your life?)
  - *I want to be active with my children and grandchildren as they're growing up.*
  - *I want to be able to help my loved one for years to come.*

Now it's your turn:
- Select a goal that is specific and challenging but not impossible
  - *I will* _____
    _____
    _____

- Ask for support from someone who can hold you accountable
  - *I will ask* _____
    _____
    _____

- Anticipate barriers and consider ways to overcome them
  - *If* _____ *, I will* _____
    _____

- Remember WHY you're setting this goal (How does doing the activity relate to what's important in your life?)
  - *I want to* _____ *because I* _____
    _____

Appendix D

ADVOCATING TO FIGHT STIGMA AND DISCRIMINATION

LOVING SOMEONE WHO HAS A MENTAL ILLNESS can take a great deal of time and emotion, and sometimes just getting through the day can be difficult. If you are so inclined and have the time and energy, you may want to fight stigma and discrimination in ways that feel right to you. Even if getting involved in formal advocacy efforts does not suit you, you can do small things in your own relationships and community that make a difference . . . and doing so can feel empowering and meaningful.

As noted in chapter 4, there are many ways to fight stigma and discrimination. One of the most impactful strategies is through personal connections. Therefore, **consider sharing your story**. Your loved one may wish to talk about their experiences as well. Although doing so can feel vulnerable, first-hand accounts of mental illness can educate, instill empathy, reduce fear, and changes attitudes. Many popular actors (Kristen Bell, Wayne Brady, Matthew Perry), musicians (Lil Wayne, James Taylor, Lizzo, Selena Gomez), and athletes (Naomi Osaka, Simone Biles, DeMar DeRozan) are publicly sharing their experience of mental illness or substance misuse and getting therapy. Hopefully, their openness can decrease stigma and encourage others to seek help.

In addition to sharing your story, you can publicly express your perspectives related to mental health via **social media, blogs, and letters to the editor**. You can follow the legislature and **contact your state representatives** to relate your experience and encourage them to support mental health bills; personal stories can be quite persuasive for elected officials.

Another advocacy opportunity is to **give feedback when you encounter stigma-tizing messages**, either in the media or in everyday conversation. You may name how the communication or behavior contributes to stigma surrounding mental illness. You can provide facts and reputable resources where people can learn more (see Resource List for websites of trustworthy organizations). You may share your emotional reaction as well, noting how you feel hurt or angry. It's helpful to deliver this information in a non-attacking manner, presuming that the misinformation or negative portrayal was based on a lack of education rather than any negative intent.

Finally, consider using and encouraging others to **use "people-first language."** Instead of referring to people by their diagnosis (such as schizophrenic or borderline), use words such as a person "has schizophrenia" or is "living with borderline personality disorder." This approach puts the person before the illness, demonstrates respect, and can contribute to decreasing stigma. Mental illness is just one part of your loved one, and it's not appropriate to define them by a label. Your loved one has many other parts of their identity—perhaps they are an amazing cook, have a wonderful sense of humor, are great mechanical engineers, or are playful with children. The words you use matter.

Organizations Working to Eliminate Stigma and Discrimination

Many organizations are actively working to end stigma and discrimination surrounding mental illness. Groups are trying to make it OK to talk openly about mental health by creating media campaigns, community events, school-based educational sessions, and support programs. You may get some helpful ideas and feel a sense of hope by looking at these organizations' websites. Speaking out against stigma and discrimination and being part of larger advocacy efforts can help many people. If you're interested, you could contact one of these organizations.

ORGANIZATION	DESCRIPTION	WEBSITE
National Alliance on Mental Illness (NAMI)	This grassroots mental health organization provides educational classes and support groups and advocates for change in mental health care. Over 600 affiliates are located across the United States. Read more about NAMI in chapter 3.	www.nami.org
Depression and Bipolar Alliance (DBSA)	As a national organization focuses on depression and bipolar disorder, it offers 450 peer-based, wellness-oriented support groups across the United States, both in person and virtually; it also has training programs for peer support specialists.	www.dbsalliance.org
Bring Change to Mind (BC2M)	Founded by the actress Glenn Close after her sister was diagnosed with bipolar disorder and her nephew with schizoaffective disorder, it offers workshops for youth and multimedia campaigns to spark open dialogue and put an end to stigma surrounding mental illness.	www.bringchange2mind.org
"Make it OK" campaign	This Minnesota-based campaign encourages conversations about mental illness through podcasts and an interactive website which includes quizzes to identify stigma, real-life examples of stigma, and an opportunity to pledge to stop stigma.	www.makeitok.org
Born this Way Foundation	Founded by Lady Gaga and her mother, it encourages people to practice kindness to themselves and others. It offers in-person and online programs and campaigns to support open discussion about mental health.	www.bornthisway. foundation
Stamp Out Stigma	Sponsored by the Association for Behavioral Health and Wellness, it encourages people to take a pledge to work toward the three Rs: Recognizing the illnesses, Re-educating ourselves and others, and Reducing stigma.	www.stampoutstigma.com

ORGANIZATION	DESCRIPTION	WEBSITE
Boris Lawrence Henson Foundation	It strives to eliminate stigma in the African American community via awareness campaigns, provision of referrals for mental health resources, and scholarships to Black students seeking careers in the mental health field.	www.borislhensonfoundation.org
Melanin & Mental Health	It encourages Black and Latinx communities to seek mental health support. The website includes resources, learning opportunities, and a therapist directory.	www.melaninandmentalhealth.com
The Confess Project	It empowers barbers to be mental health advocates in order to build a culture of mental health for Black youth, men, and their families.	www.theconfessproject.com
Asian Mental Health Collective	It centers on combating stigma in the Asian community. The website includes a therapist directory, personal stories, and information about community events.	www.asianmhc.org
Indian Health Service's Suicide Prevention and Care Program	This national initiative addresses suicide prevention among American Indian and Alaska Native communities and promotes collaboration among tribes, tribal organizations, and the Indian Health Service.	www.ihs.gov/suicideprevention
Depression Looks Like Me	It specifically addresses stigma surrounding mental illness among LGBTQ+ individuals.	www.depressionlookslikeme.com
Treatment Advocacy Center	It strives to increase access to treatment for people with serious mental illness by promoting laws and practices that eliminate barriers to care.	www.treatmentadvocacycenter.org

ORGANIZATION	DESCRIPTION	WEBSITE
Schizophrenia and Psychosis Action Alliance	It focuses on creating systemic change to improve equity, care, and support for people with schizophrenia and other psychotic disorders.	www.sczaction.org
National Shattering Silence Coalition	It works to make policy reforms to ensure people with "serious brain disorders receive equitable, compassionate, and collaborative treatment and support."	www.nationalshattering-silencecoalition.org
The Mental Health Coalition	This coalition of organizations is united to end stigma surrounding mental illness, with special emphasis on BIPOC, black, AAPI and LGBTQ communities.	www.thementalhealthcoalition.org

Appendix E

MENTAL HEALTH PROFESSIONALS, SERVICES, AND SUPPORT GROUPS

MANY PEOPLE PARTICIPATE IN MENTAL HEALTH services every year. Research by the Centers for Disease Control and Prevention (CDC) found that 20% of adults had received mental health treatment the preceding year, including 17% who had taken mental health medication and 10% who had received therapy from a mental health professional.[78]

Many effective treatments exist to help people living with a mental illness. However, insurance coverage and access to programs can vary considerably, often with fewer services and longer waiting lists in rural areas. It can be helpful to contact your insurance company to understand your benefits and which providers, clinics, and services are covered under your plan. If your loved one does not have insurance, some federal funded health centers, county programs, and university counseling centers offer free or low-cost services.

This Appendix provides an overview of

- Training and roles of different mental health professionals

- Types of mental health services

- Additional options: Mobile apps and complementary and alternative medicine

- Types of peer support groups and classes

Mental Health Professionals

Providers who prescribe medications

Psychiatrists are physicians (MD or DO) with special training in treating mental illness. After the initial assessment, subsequent sessions are usually brief and focus on the medications and side effects. Although some psychiatrists provide psychotherapy as part of their visits, many refer clients to other providers for additional services.

Psychiatric-mental health (PMH) nurses have nursing degrees (RN, APRN, DPN) with specialized training in treating mental illness.

Psychiatric pharmacists (PharmD) can prescribe medications in some, but not all, states. They have special training in mental health medications, including dosing, side effects, and drug interactions.

Primary care providers ("general practitioners") prescribe medications for many mental health conditions. These providers can also continue a medication plan that has been started by a specialist once the client has stabilized. Primary care providers can be physicians, advanced care nurses, or physician assistants (PA).

Providers who focus on psychotherapy and/or testing

Psychologists (PhD or PsyD) have a doctoral degree and specific skills in both psychological testing and talk therapy, including individual, group, couples, and family counseling. Although some psychologists (often those living in rural areas) can prescribe some mental health medications, most do not.

Social workers (BSW, MSW, DSW) have a bachelors, masters, or doctoral degree and work in a variety of settings such as schools, clinics, hospitals, hospice, military, and prisons. Many social workers provide counseling, and they often have strong skills in connecting clients with community resources, such as help with accessing housing, insurance, benefits, and emergency resources.

Marriage and family therapists (MFT) have graduate training in working specifically with couples and families. They focus on the family system, thinking about the client within their family relationships. They often involve partners, parents, and children in treatment.

Many other professionals provide therapy as well, such as pastoral counselors, licensed professional counselors (LPC), and addiction counselors. In addition, professionals from other disciplines often play key roles in comprehensive mental health treatment programs, such as case managers, recreation therapists, dietitians, and occupational therapists.

Let's now review some different kinds of mental health services.

Mental Health Services

Although each service is listed separately, many people utilize several treatment options at the same time.

Counseling and testing (psychological services): Psychological services include psycho-therapy (individual, couples, family, or group counseling), psychological testing, classes, and workshops. A wide variety of mental health professionals provide counseling (see previous section). Chapter 7 offers tips on how to select a therapist.

Counseling is provided in many different settings, but most people first access therapy in the outpatient setting, such as a mental health clinic. Frequency of outpatient services varies, but a weekly format is common. Mental health services address a wide range of topics, including improving wellness, getting the most from medications, and learning about the illness. People can also learn skills, such as getting along with others, setting and working toward goals, solving problems, reducing or eliminating use of substances, getting more involved in enjoyable activities, communicating effectively, and managing stress and anxiety.

Although many counseling models exist, cognitive-behavioral therapy (CBT) approaches are the most commonly used treatments and have the strongest research base. Acceptance and Commitment Therapy (ACT), a newer model of therapy that incorporates mindfulness and a focus on psychological flexibility, has also been found to be effective in treating depression, anxiety, and substance misuse.[79] Some individual therapy approaches for specific mental illnesses have strong research support, such as cognitive behavioral therapy for psychosis (CBTp),[80] interpersonal and social rhythm therapy for bipolar disorder,[81] and both CBT[82] and interpersonal therapy[83] for major depression.

Psychological testing (assessment) is typically conducted by psychologists. Testing can be especially useful when the mental health diagnosis is unclear. Assessment reports not only provide the test results and diagnostic conclusions, but also contain recommendations for the treatment plan.

Medication management (psychiatry services): Psychiatric providers make clinical diagnoses and are able to prescribe medications and other treatments for mental illness. The first session is generally an assessment, and follow-up appointments typically occur every one to three months; ongoing appointments are generally brief (15–20 minutes) and tend to focus on medication effectiveness and side effects. Of note, many kinds of professionals prescribe mental health medications (see listing of mental health professionals in preceding section).

Telehealth Services

Many of the services described in this appendix are offered both in-person and via telehealth. The COVID pandemic led to a significant increase in telemedicine services for mental health problems,[85] especially for psychotherapy and psychiatry appointments. Telehealth services can be delivered in a variety of modes such as video, telephone, text messaging, and more.

Research has documented high levels of patient satisfaction with telehealth, including flexibility, ease of access, decreased travel time (which can be especially helpful for rural individuals), comfort of services in one's own home, and a smaller time commitment.[86] Further, video-based telehealth has been found to be as effective, if not more, than in-person care for mental health problems.[87]

It's important for people to have the option of where they would like to receive their mental health care. Some may prefer in-person sessions if they lack privacy at home, do not have reliable internet access, feel a more personal connection with the provider when in person, or have concerns about the hassles and security of telehealth interactions.

Thus, as you explore treatment options for your loved one and yourself, consider your preferences for telehealth versus in person. You may also want to check with your insurance company to see if there are any differences in coverage and costs for telehealth services.

Electroconvulsive therapy (ECT): This treatment, also provided by psychiatrists, has been available for many years and can yield rapid improvements in symptoms associated with severe depression and bipolar disorder. ECT is performed under general anesthesia and involves inducing a brief seizure; most people have multiple treatments over time. Stigma remains about ECT due to media misrepresentation and the manner in which the treatment was historically delivered; however, the current mode of delivery is safe, and the treatment is generally quite well tolerated.

"Treatment resistant" therapies: Psychiatrists may recommend these newer treatments when first-line medications and therapies don't yield satisfactory results. The medication ketamine, vagus nerve stimulation (VNS), and repetitive transcranial magnetic stimulation (rTMS) are growing in popularity and, although preliminary, have promising outcomes to date.

Peer support: As discussed in chapter 6, peer support specialists are people with lived experience of mental illness who receive formal training in helping others. Peer support can be provided in several settings such as clubhouses, mental health clinics, hospitals, jails, and prisons. Specialists are also integrated into interprofessional teams such as Assertive Community Treatment (ACT) teams and crisis response teams. Specialists draw upon and share their own recovery experience as they help people learn skills, manage crises, access health care, advocate for services, and develop recovery plans. Peer specialists can be empowering role models and friends for those in the throes of difficult times.

Case management: Case managers work with people in setting and working toward goals, connecting with community resources and services, and managing crises. Case managers can serve as important advocates as they facilitate coordination among providers and services.

Coaching (supported employment, academic support): These services help people enjoy and succeed in important aspects of their lives. Job coaches assist people in managing anxiety and on-the-job stress and can work with employers on helpful accommodations. One model of supported employment with strong research support, Individual Placement and Support, helps people select and succeed in competitive jobs. Coaches help with developing a resume, preparing for interviews, and performing well on the job.[84] Other types of coaches provide support in school (academic coaching) and the community (life skills coaches who help with bills, appointments, shopping, etc.). Availability and insurance coverage vary considerably for these services.

Clubhouse (community resource center): Clubhouses are community centers that provide many programs and services for people with a mental illness. Individualized plans are developed, and members are supported with their recovery goals such as finding housing, landing a job, or getting additional training. Grounded in a spirit of peer support, hope, mutual respect, and empowerment, clubhouses provide a sense of belonging, meaningful relationships, social activities, and access to crisis services when needed. To find a clubhouse in your area, see the Clubhouse International website (www.clubhouse-intl.org).

Assertive community treatment teams: ACT teams typically include one professional who prescribes medication as well as case managers, therapists, and peer specialists. Teams visit people at home and offer support with activities of daily living, such as shopping and paying bills, medication management, and preventing crises. ACT teams also assist people in creating routines filled with meaningful activities. Family members are often encouraged to work collaboratively with ACT team members in support of their loved one.

Partial hospitalization program (PHP), Intensive outpatient program (IOP), or day treatment program: These programs may be a step-down from an inpatient or residential program or may be a way to prevent an inpatient stay. Although programs vary in their approach, many offer four to eight hours of classes, therapy, and group sessions, which occur several days per week, as well as regular contact with a medication provider. People may live at home, at a halfway house, or at a sober living facility while participating. Although focused on the person with the mental illness, many programs offer opportunities for family participation.

Short-term stabilization (hospitalization): The goal of an inpatient admission is typically de-escalation of the acute crisis and creation of a discharge plan to help the client continue to stabilize and progress. The average length of hospital stay is generally quite short, often due to insurance restrictions. Family members and friends can provide invaluable information to the treatment team during this time.

Residential treatment: Some people benefit from a longer period of 24/7 support than can be provided on an inpatient unit. Some insurance plans cover one to three months in residential treatment centers; this allows for more time to stabilize the crisis, build skills, and develop a robust aftercare plan.

Crisis services: When a mental health emergency arises, people usually get care in an emergency room, crisis center, or legal setting. People are evaluated by a team of professionals who then make recommendations. Depending on the nature of the crisis, the treatment plan may be "voluntary" or "involuntary."

A *"voluntary admission"* occurs when the individual desires and consents to inpatient treatment. This process can get off to a good start because the individual recognizes the need for and wants help.

"Involuntary admission" (commitment) laws vary by state, so it's helpful to familiarize yourself with your local statues and standards. Generally, people can be committed if they are in an acute crisis and deemed not able to make decisions about their own well-being. Common reasons for involuntary commitment include being a danger to oneself or others, acutely psychotic, or unable to care for themselves. These situations can be tricky and controversial as health care providers balance the person's need for immediate help with their civil rights.

Generally, a "72-hour hold" (also known as "psychiatric hold") is used when there is an urgent need for psychiatric evaluation. Afterwards, a judge can order someone to continue treatment in the hospital ("inpatient civil commitment" or "involuntary hospitalization") or in the community ("outpatient civil commitment"—also known as "assisted outpatient treatment").

Coordinated Specialty Care Programs ("First Episode Programs") for Schizophrenia

Coordinated Specialty Care Programs (or "first episode psychosis programs") are model programs that integrate many treatment approaches into a comprehensive package. Created specifically for people who are just starting to have symptoms of schizophrenia, the goals are to identify symptoms as early as possible, engage the client and family into care from the beginning, and improve the course of the illness over time.

These services are individualized and involve a team of providers who offer medication management, job or education supports, counseling, and family education. All of these pieces work together to strengthen resiliency and the ability to manage symptoms. Research has found that participation in these programs is related to a better quality of life, feeling more empowered, greater independence, improved functioning in school or work, and lower rates of relapse.[88]

As with many mental health services, access to these services varies widely across the country; you can search for available programs in your state on the Substance Abuse and Mental Health Services Administration website (https://www.samhsa.gov/esmi-treatment-locator).

Additional Options: Mobile Apps and Complementary and Alternative Medicine

Two other options that are growing in popularity include mobile apps and complementary and alternative medicine.

Mobile apps: Many mobile apps have been developed for mental health issues, and most are free or low-cost. The quality can vary considerably, and generally apps are best as a supplement to professional care rather than as a replacement. You may wish to check the One Mind website (www.onemindpsyberguide.org) to find various apps for different mental health issues; this website also includes professional assessments of the apps' credibility, user experience, and privacy policies.

Complementary and alternative medicine: Consistent with the "whole-person care" approach to recovery, these products or practices can address mind, body, and spirit. They may include physical therapies such as yoga, meditation, massage, bright lights, or acupuncture; vitamins and minerals; and herbal remedies such as St John's wort and homeopathy. Although some of these therapies show promise, many have not yet been thoroughly tested. Also, some can have side effects and interact with other medications. It's important to talk openly with your health care provider if using these therapies.

Now that we have reviewed different types of mental health providers and an array of mental health treatments, the final section of this appendix describes peer support programs.

Peer Support Groups and Classes

Peer support groups are an excellent way for people living with a mental illness or substance misuse problem to connect and learn from others with similar experiences. For example, Alcoholics Anonymous (AA) is an international 12-step program for people managing concerns with alcohol use that has existed since 1935.

Many support groups and classes are available, including programs focused on mental illness such as the NAMI Peer-to-Peer educational program described in chapter 3. Across all of these programs, people with shared life experiences come together to

- Listen without judgment

- Give and receive encouragement

- Extend hope

- Share skills and resources

- Offer friendship

Support groups listed in this table are all free. Many organizations have both virtual and in-person meetings.

Note: There are thousands of groups around the world, and the norms vary considerably across programs. Some groups convey the viewpoint that mental health medications are not appropriate for people in recovery. If this sentiment is expressed, we encourage you to consider finding another meeting as that stance is not universally held and is not consistent with the science of recovery.

PEER SUPPORT GROUPS

Mental Health Condition	Name	Description	Website
All mental illnesses	NAMI (National Alliance on Mental Illness) Connection Recovery Support Group	90-minute, confidential support groups for adults (18+) with mental health conditions	www.nami.org
Depression and bipolar disorder	Depression and Bipolar Support Alliance (DBSA)	Support groups for people with depression or bipolar disorder and those who love them	www.dbsalliance.org
Alcohol misuse	Alcoholics Anonymous (AA)	12-step support groups for anyone who would like support with their drinking problem	www.aa.org
Narcotic use	Narcotics Anonymous (NA)	12-step support groups for people for whom drugs have become a considerable problem	www.na.org
Mental illness and substance misuse	Dual Recovery Anonymous (DRA)	12-step programs for people with substance misuse and mental illness	www.draonline.org
Any addiction	Self-Management and Recovery Training—SMART Recovery	Structured support meetings grounded in scientific evidence about how people can move away from addiction and make choices that foster greater self-regard	www.smartrecovery.org
Any addiction	Celebrate Recovery	Christian 12-step support groups for anyone dealing with hurt, pain, or addiction of any kind	www.celebraterecovery.com

Appendix F

FAMILY EDUCATION PROGRAMS AND SUPPORT GROUPS

THIS APPENDIX DESCRIBES TWO TYPES of services for family members and friends:

- Family education programs
- Family support groups

Family Education Programs

These free courses offer information about mental illness, coping tools, tips on how to set limits, and empowerment as you advocate for your loved one. Most programs involve structured, time-limited classes with set curricula, and are led (or co-led) by trained family members with lived experience. These classes offer opportunities to learn from other families managing similar situations, which can be comforting.

Of note, the programs listed in this table are offered only for family members and friends. The person with the mental illness does not attend, which allows participants to speak freely without censoring or worrying about hurting their loved one's feelings.

FAMILY EDUCATION COURSES

Mental Health Condition	Name	Description	Website
All mental illnesses	Family to Family Program (National Alliance on Mental Illness, NAMI)	8-session educational program including group discussion, presentations, and activities (see chapter 3 for more information about NAMI)	www.nami.org
All mental illnesses	Mental Health First Aid (MHFA) (National Council for Mental Wellbeing)	1-day class that educates and offers skills for recognizing and dealing with mental health and substance use crises	www.mentalhealthfirstaid.org
All mental illness including PTSD (military)	NAMI Homefront	6-session educational course for adults who care about a veteran/ service member with a mental illness including PTSD	www.nami.org
All mental illnesses (with focus on PTSD)	Support And Family Education (SAFE) Program	18-session course created in the VA system, addressing all mental illnesses but with special emphasis on trauma/PTSD	www.ouhsc.edu/SafeProgram
Borderline Personality Disorder (BPD)	Family Connections (National Education Alliance for Borderline Personality Disorder)	12-session course including education, support, and skills training	www.borderline-personalitydisorder.org/family-connections/

Family Support Groups

The following support groups for family members and friends are also offered at no charge. Meetings are available on an ongoing basis, allowing for the development of friendships and mutual support over time. Led (or co-led) by peers or trained family members with lived experience, these groups usually have general goals but do not follow a set curriculum. The loved one with the illness does not attend these groups. Many organizations have both virtual and in-person meetings.

FAMILY PEER SUPPORT GROUPS

Mental Health Condition	Name	Description	Website
All mental illnesses	Family Support Group (National Alliance on Mental Illness, NAMI)	60- to 90-minute support groups for adults (18+) with a loved one who has mental health problems (see chapter 3 for more information about NAMI)	www.nami.org
Depression and bipolar disorder	Depression and Bipolar Support Alliance (DBSA)	Support groups for people with depression or bipolar disorder and those that love them	www.dbsalliance.org
Alcohol misuse and drug use	Al-Anon* and Nar-Anon	12-step support groups for adults who care about someone managing an alcohol (Al-Anon) or drug problem (Nar-Anon)	www.al-anon.org (alcohol) www.nar-anon.org (drugs) www.familiesanonymous.org (alcohol or drugs)
Alcohol misuse and drug use	Alateen and Narateen	12-step support groups for teenagers who care about someone who has an alcohol (Alateen) or drug problem (Narateen)	www.al-anon.org/newcomers/teen-corner-alateen/ www.nar-anon.org/narateen

FAMILY PEER SUPPORT GROUPS			
Mental Health Condition	Name	Description	Website
Any addiction	Self-Management and Recovery Training—SMART Recovery: Family and Friends	Structured support meetings for friends and family members of people engaging in addictive behavior that teaches tools grounded in cognitive behavioral theory	www.smartrecovery.org
Alcohol misuse and drug use	Community Reinforcement Approach to Family Training (CRAFT)-Helping Families Help	Ongoing groups for friends and families whose loved one has problems with alcohol or drugs that focus on communication skills, empathy, accessing treatment, allowing for natural consequences, and setting boundaries	www.helpingfamilieshelp.com/groups-for-families

* Al-Anon also has a free mobile app through which you can connect with others and offer mutual support via electronic meetings and private chats (www.al-anon.org/for-members/members-resources/mobile-app/).

RESOURCE LIST

Trustworthy Information on Mental Illness, PTSD, and Substance Misuse

Nonprofit Organizations

National Alliance on Mental Illness (NAMI): www.nami.org

Depression and Bipolar Support Alliance (DBSA): www.dbsalliance.org

Mental Health America: www.mhanational.org

Anxiety and Depression Association of America: www.adaa.org

American Foundation for Suicide Prevention: www.afsp.org

Treatment Advocacy Center: www.treatmentadvocacycenter.org

Professional Organizations

American Psychological Association: www.apa.org/topics

American Psychiatric Association—Patients and Families Section: www.psychiatry.org/patients-families

La Salud Mental: www.psychiatry.org/patients-families/la-salud-mental
Information for Spanish speaking patients and families

Federal Agencies

Substance Abuse and Mental Health Services Administration (SAMHSA): www.samhsa.gov

- Has 24/7 anonymous information service that provides referrals to local support groups, treatment facilities, and community organizations, including first-episode psychosis programs (1-800-662-HELP and www.findtreatment.gov)

National Institute for Mental Health: www.nimh.nih.gov

National Center for PTSD: www.ptsd.va.gov
Includes several free mobile apps including PTSD Family Coach for adults who love someone who has PTSD

Other

Center for Practice Innovation (CPI): www.practiceinnovations.org/resources
Consumer and Family Portal has many videos by consumers and family members hosted by the Columbia Psychiatry New York State Psychiatric Institute

PsychCentral: www.psychcentral.com

National Resource Center on Psychiatric Advance Directives: www.nrc-pad.org

The Care Hack: www.thecarehack.com
Online program for caregivers of people living with a mental illness, focusing on actionable content, coaching, and building community

International Resources

Head to Head (Australia): www.headtohealth.gov.au

Canadian Mental Health Association: www.cmha.ca

Mood Disorders Society of Canada: www.mdsc.ca

Mental Health Foundation (United Kingdom): www.mentalhealth.org.uk

Mind (England and Wales): www.mind.org.uk

Hotlines (all offer free, confidential 24/7 support)

Suicide and Crisis Lifeline: www.suicidepreventionlifeline.org
988—call or text with a trained counselor; can also use chat services via website

- **Veterans:** Select option 1 (or chat via website: www.veteranscrisisline.net)

- **En Espanol:** Select option 2

- **American Sign Language:** Available via an interpreter on the website and videophone

Trevor Project: www.thetrevorproject.org
Suicide prevention and crisis intervention for LGBTQ (lesbian, gay, bisexual, transgender, queer, and questioning) young people
866-488-7386

LGBT National Hotline: www.lgbthotline.org
888-843-4564

Trans Lifeline: www.translifeline.org
877-565-8860 (USA); 877-330-6366 (Canada)

National Domestic Violence Hotline: www.thehotline.org
800-799-7233 (SAFE) or text "start" to 88788
Has advocates available who can help access shelters and treatment

National Sexual Assault Hotline: www.rainn.org
800-656-HOPE (4673)
Operated by RAINN (Rape, Abuse & Incest National Network) and also has a free mobile app

National Child Abuse Hotline: www.childhelp.org
800-4-A-CHILD (422-4453)

ACKNOWLEDGMENTS

OUR SINCERE GRATITUDE TO

Our early readers who gave us the green light of encouragement, acknowledging the need for such a book, validating our tone and approach, and urging us to keep writing.

Our reviewers, namely friends and colleagues who love people with a mental illness, as well as those with lived experience of mental illness or PTSD themselves. Your insightful, heartfelt feedback and your permission to include your stories made this book more relatable and personal.

Advocates Marilyn Dornfeld and Mindy Greiling who provided detailed, astute feedback. Your insights and wisdom shaped by your family experiences, years of teaching National Alliance on Mental Illness classes, and advocacy and legislative activity, helped us stay grounded in the real-world experience of families and supported us in delicately navigating controversial topics.

The clinical experts in the trenches who reviewed sections and provided excellent recommendations. Specifically, we thank Shirley Glynn, PhD, clinical psychologist at the University of California, Los Angeles, and national expert in family involvement in the treatment of serious mental illness and PTSD. Your invaluable, wise feedback on the entire book helped make it as accurate, accessible, and useful as possible.

The entire team at Johns Hopkins University Press who shepherded our book through the publication process. James Monroe whose artistic illustrations help convey our message so well. Paul Payson who provided superior and thoughtful copy editing. Chanel Copeland, PA-C MHS, faculty at Duke University, who served as a cultural sensitivity reader.

The individuals, couples, and families that trusted me (Michelle) as your psychologist. It has been a privilege to work with and learn from you. Thank you for sharing your story; allowing me to witness your pain, courage, resilience, and strength; and letting me be part of your journey.

And for those dear to us . . . Dudley, our father and husband, whose continued encouragement, patience, and assistance with the innumerable aspects of writing books have been deeply appreciated; thank you for your tremendous support! Noah, our nephew and grandson whose insightful feedback helped us recognize critical concepts that needed further explanation. Your perspectives as a 20-year-old male were so important and truly improved many sections of our book. Lisa, our brilliant sister and daughter who believed in this book and has been our most passionate cheerleader from the very beginning. Your energy and enthusiasm fueled us, and your wise, detailed feedback shows up on every page. Grand merci.

In the spirit of self-reflexivity, we acknowledge that we authors are white, cisgender women living in the midwestern region of the United States, both of whom manage some physical disabilities and both of whom love several people living with a mental illness. Our knowledge is deeply rooted in our personal lives as well as Michelle's 30 years of experience conducting psychotherapy, developing family education programs, and doing research. In writing this book, we have intentionally elicited reviews and detailed feedback from a variety of readers who represent considerable diversity across many domains. We have worked hard to address our biases and make our book accessible and meaningful to a diverse readership. We acknowledge that our privilege and positionality influenced our writing.

NOTES

1 Pennebaker, J. W., & Smyth, J. M. (2016). *Opening up by writing it down: How expressive writing improves health and eases emotional pain.* Guilford Press.

2 Ringeisen, H., Edlund, M., Guyer, H., Geiger, P., Stambaugh, L., Dever, J., Liao, D., Carr, C., Peytchev, A., Reed, W., McDaniel, K., & Smith, T. (2023). *Mental and Substance Use Disorders Prevalence Study (MDPS): Findings Report.* RTI International; Substance Abuse and Mental Health Services Administration. (2021). *Key substance use and mental health indicators in the United States: Results from the 2020 National Survey on Drug Use and Health* (HHS Publication No. PEP21-07-01-003, NSDUH Series H-56).

3 Mennano, J. [@thesecurerelationship]. (2024, April 8). *Only when we can access our feelings, sit with them, name them, and make sense of them, can we ever* [Post]. Instagram. www.instagram.com/p/CqzMGOVLK1r.

4 Ponte, K. (2020). *ForLikeMinds: Mental illness recovery insights.* Real MH Works.

5 Åsbø, G., Ueland, T., Haatveit, B., Bjella, T., Flaaten, C. B., Wold, K. F., . . . & Simonsen, C. (2022). The time is ripe for a consensus definition of clinical recovery in first-episode psychosis: Suggestions based on a 10-year follow-up study. *Schizophrenia Bulletin, 48*(4), 839–849; Kelly, K. M., & Mezuk, B. (2017). Predictors of remission from generalized anxiety disorder and major depressive disorder. *Journal of Affective Disorders, 208,* 467–474.

6 Fekadu, W., Mihiretu, A., Craig, T. K., & Fekadu, A. (2019). Multidimensional impact of severe mental illness on family members: Systematic review. *BMJ Open, 9*(12), e032391.

7 Lucksted, A., Medoff, D., Burland, J., Stewart, B., Fang, L. J., Brown, C., Jones, A., Lehman, A., & Dixon, L. B. (2013). Sustained outcomes of a peer-taught family education program on mental illness. *Acta Psychiatrica Scandinavica, 127*(4), 279–286; Mercado, M., Fuss, A. A., Sawano, N., Gensemer, A., Brennan, W., McManus, K., Dixon, L., Haselden, M., & Cleek, A. F. (2016). Generalizability of the NAMI family-to-family education program: Evidence from an efficacy study. *Psychiatric Services, 67*(6), 591–593.

8 Piercy, K. L., Troiano, R. P., Ballard, R. M., Carlson, S. A., Fulton, J. E., Galuska, D. A., George, S., & Olson, R. D. (2018). The physical activity guidelines for Americans. *Journal of the American Medical Association, 320*(19), 2020–2028.

9 Garcia, L., Pearce, M., Abbas, A., Mok, A., Strain, T., Ali, S., Crippa, A., Dempsey, P., Golubic, R., Kelly, P., Laird, Y., McNamara, E., Moore, S., Herick de Sa, T., Smith, A., Wijndaele, K., Woodcock, J., & Brage, S. (2023). Non-occupational physical activity and risk of cardiovascular disease, cancer and mortality outcomes: A dose–response meta-analysis of large prospective studies. *British Journal of Sports Medicine, 57*(15), 979–989.

10 Singh, B., Olds, T., Curtis, R., Dumuid, D., Virgara, R., Watson, A., Szeto, K., O'Connor, E., Ferguson, T., Eglitis, E., Miatke, A., Simpson, C., & Maher, C. (2023). Effectiveness of physical activity interventions for improving depression, anxiety and distress: An overview of systematic reviews. *British Journal of Sports Medicine, 57*(18), 1203–1209.

11 Wicks, C., Barton, J., Orbell, S., & Andrews, L. (2022). Psychological benefits of outdoor physical activity in natural versus urban environments: A systematic review and meta-analysis of experimental studies. *Applied Psychology: Health and Well-Being, 14*(3), 1037–1061.

12 Hoge, E. A., Bui, E., Mete, M., Dutton, M. A., Baker, A. W., & Simon, N. M. (2023). Mindfulness-based stress reduction vs escitalopram for the treatment of adults with anxiety disorders: A randomized clinical trial. *Journal of the American Medical Association Psychiatry, 80*(1), 13–21; Schlechta Portella, C. F., Ghelman, R., Abdala, V., Schveitzer, M. C., & Afonso, R. F. (2021). Meditation: Evidence map of systematic reviews. *Frontiers in Public Health, 9*, 1777.

13 Ford, B. Q., Lam, P., John, O. P., & Mauss, I. B. (2018). The psychological health benefits of accepting negative emotions and thoughts: Laboratory, diary, and longitudinal evidence. *Journal of Personality and Social Psychology, 115*(6), 1075.

14 Neff, K. D. (2023). Self-compassion: Theory, method, research, and intervention. *Annual Review of Psychology, 74*, 193–218.

15 Radmacher, M. (2009). *Courage doesn't always roar.* Conari Press.

16 Holt-Lunstad, J., Smith, T. B., Baker, M., Harris, T., & Stephenson, D. (2015). Loneliness and social isolation as risk factors for mortality: A meta-analytic review. *Perspectives on Psychological Science, 10*(2), 227–237.

17 Kemp, A.H., Arias, J.A., & Fisher, Z. (2017). Social ties, health and wellbeing: A literature review and model. In A. Ibáñez, L. Sedeño, & A. García (Eds), *Neuroscience and social science: The missing link* (pp. 397-427) Springer; Leigh-Hunt, N., Bagguley, D., Bash, K., Turner, V., Turnbull, S., Valtorta, N., & Caan, W. (2017). An overview of systematic reviews on the public health consequences of social isolation and loneliness. *Public Health, 152*, 157–171.

18 Holt-Lunstad, J., Robles, T. F., & Sbarra, D. A. (2017). Advancing social connection as a public health priority in the United States. *American Psychologist, 72*(6), 517–530.

19 Dixon, L. B., Lucksted, A., Medoff, D. R., Burland, J., Stewart, B., Lehman, A. F., Fang, L., Sturm, V., Brown, C., &Murray-Swank, A. (2011). Outcomes of a randomized study of a peer-taught family-to-family education program for mental illness. *Psychiatric Services, 62*(6), 591–597.

20 Duckworth, K. (2022). *You are not alone: The NAMI guide to navigating mental health with advice from experts and wisdom from real people and families.* Zando.

21 Corrigan, P. W., Druss, B. G., & Perlick, D. A. (2014). The impact of mental illness stigma on seeking and participating in mental health care. *Psychological Science in the Public Interest, 15*(2), 37–70.

22 Corrigan, P. W., & Rao, D. (2012). On the self-stigma of mental illness: Stages, disclosure, and strategies for change. *The Canadian Journal of Psychiatry, 57*(8), 464–469.

23 Ringeisen, H., Edlund, M., Guyer, H., Geiger, P., Stambaugh, L., Dever, J., Liao, D., Carr, C., Peytchev, A., Reed, W., McDaniel, K., & Smith, T. (2023). *Mental and Substance Use Disorders Prevalence Study (MDPS): Findings Report.* RTI International; Substance Abuse and Mental Health Services Administration. (2021). *Key substance use and mental health indicators in the United States: Results from the 2020 National Survey on Drug Use and Health* (HHS Publication No. PEP21-07-01-003, NSDUH Series H-56).

24 Pescosolido, B. A., Halpern-Manners, A., Luo, L., & Perry, B. (2021). Trends in public stigma of mental illness in the US, 1996–2018. *JAMA Network Open, 4*(12), e2140202–e2140202.

25 Bhushan, D. (2022, August 26). Op-Ed: I am California's acting surgeon general. And I have bipolar disorder. *Los Angeles Times.* www.latimes.com/opinion/story/2022-08-26/california-surgeon-general-bipolar-disorder-mental-health

26 Bono, G., & Sender, J. T. (2018). How gratitude connects humans to the best in themselves and in others. *Research in Human Development, 15*(3–4), 224–237.

27 Brown, B. (2018). *Dare to lead: Brave work. Tough conversations. Whole hearts.* Random House.

28 Boss, P. (2000). *Ambiguous loss: Learning to live with unresolved grief.* Harvard University Press.

29 Substance Abuse and Mental Health Services Administration. (2012). *What's recovery? SAMHSA's working definition.* Publication No PEP12-RECDEF. Retrieved from https://store.samhsa.gov/product/SAMHSA-s-Working-Definition-of-Recovery/PEP12-RECDEF.

30 Ponte, K. (2020). *ForLikeMinds: Mental illness recovery insights.* Real MH Works.

31 Mueser, K. T., Meyer, P. S., Penn, D. L., Clancy, R., Clancy, D. M., & Salyers, M. P. (2006). The Illness Management and Recovery program: Rationale, development, and preliminary findings. *Schizophrenia Bulletin, 32*(Suppl.1), S32–S43.

32 Bhushan, D. (2022, August 26). Op-Ed: I am California's acting Surgeon General. And I have bipolar disorder. *Los Angeles Times.* www.latimes.com/opinion/story/2022-08-26/california-surgeon-general-bipolar-disorder-mental-health; Stone, K. (2022). *Thrive with schizophrenia.*

33 Peterson, C., & Seligman, M. E. P. (2004). *Character strengths and virtues: A handbook and classification*. Oxford University Press and American Psychological Association.

34 Murthy, V. H. (2023). *Our epidemic of loneliness and isolation: The US Surgeon General's advisory on the healing effects of social connection and community*. United States Department of Health and Human Services. www.hhs.gov/sites/default/files/surgeon-general-social-connection-advisory.pdf

35 Giacco, D. (2023). Loneliness and mood disorders: Consequence, cause and/or unholy alliance?. *Current Opinion in Psychiatry, 36*(1), 47–53; Suman, A., Nehra, R., Sahoo, S., & Grover, S. (2023). Prevalence of loneliness and its correlates among patients with schizophrenia. *International Journal of Social Psychiatry, 69*(4), 906–915.

36 Holt-Lunstad, J., Smith, T. B., Baker, M., Harris, T., & Stephenson, D. (2015). Loneliness and social isolation as risk factors for mortality: A meta-analytic review. *Perspectives on Psychological Science, 10*(2), 227–237.

37 Insel, T. (2022). *Healing: Our path from mental illness to mental health*. Penguin Press.

38 Bond, G. R., Drake, R. E., & Becker, D. R. (2020). An update on individual placement and support. *World Psychiatry, 19*(3), 390–391.

39 Smit, D., Miguel, C., Vrijsen, J. N., Groeneweg, B., Spijker, J., & Cuijpers, P. (2023). The effectiveness of peer support for individuals with mental illness: Systematic review and meta-analysis. *Psychological Medicine, 53*(11), 5332–5341.

40 Piercy, K. L., Troiano, R. P., Ballard, R. M., Carlson, S. A., Fulton, J. E., Galuska, D. A., George, S., & Olson, R. D. (2018). The physical activity guidelines for Americans. Journal of the American Medical Association, 320(19), 2020–2028.

41 Singh, B., Olds, T., Curtis, R., Dumuid, D., Virgara, R., Watson, A., Szeto, K., O'Connor, E., Ferguson, T., Eglitis, E., Miatke, A., Simpson, C., & Maher, C. (2023). Effectiveness of physical activity interventions for improving depression, anxiety and distress: An overview of systematic reviews. British Journal of Sports Medicine, 57(18), 1203–1209.

42 Carr, A. (2019). Couple therapy, family therapy and systemic interventions for adult-focused problems: The current evidence base. *Journal of Family Therapy, 41*(4), 492–536; Fiorillo, A., Del Vecchio, V., Luciano, M., Sampogna, G., De Rosa, C., Malangone, C., Volpe, U., Bardicchia, F., Ciampini, G., Crocamo, C., Iapichino, S., Lampis, D., Moroni, A., Orlandi, E., Piselli, M., Pompili, E., Veltro, F., Carrà, G., & Maj, M. (2015). Efficacy of psychoeducational family intervention for bipolar I disorder: A controlled, multicentric, real-world study. *Journal of Affective Disorders, 172*, 291–299; Wittenborn, A. K., Woods, S. B., Priest, J. B., Morgan, P. C., Tseng, C. F., Huerta, P., & Edwards, C. (2022). Couple and family interventions for depressive and bipolar disorders: Evidence base update (2010–2019). *Journal of Marital and Family Therapy, 48*(1), 129–153.

43 Allen, S. (2018). The science of gratitude. John Templeton Foundation by the Greater Good Science Center at University of California Berkeley. https://ggsc.berkeley.edu/images/uploads/GGSC-JTF_White_Paper-Gratitude-FINAL.pdf

44 Algoe, S. B., Fredrickson, B. L., & Gable, S. L. (2013). The social functions of the emotion of gratitude via expression. *Emotion, 13*(4), 605–609.

45 Mennano, J. [@thesecurerelationship]. (2024, May 21). *I see you I hear you I'm safe I'm on your team I see you I hear you* [Post]. Instagram. www.instagram.com/p/CshzdZrrbXO.

46 Covey, S. (2013). *The 7 habits of highly effective people: Powerful lessons in personal change.* Simon & Schuster.

47 Hudson, T. (1999). *Compassionate caring: A daily pilgrimage of pain and hope.* Eagle.

48 Gottman, J.M. (1993). A theory of marital dissolution and stability. *Journal of Family Psychology, 7*(1), 57–75.

49 Masten, A. S., Lucke, C. M., Nelson, K. M., & Stallworthy, I. C. (2021). Resilience in development and psychopathology: Multisystem perspectives. *Annual Review of Clinical Psychology, 17,* 521–549.

50 Leen-Feldner, E. W., Feldner, M. T., Bunaciu, L., & Blumenthal, H. (2011). Associations between parental posttraumatic stress disorder and both offspring internalizing problems and parental aggression within the National Comorbidity Survey-Replication. *Journal of Anxiety Disorders, 25*(2), 169–175; Rasic, D., Hajek, T., Alda, M., & Uher, R. (2014). Risk of mental illness in offspring of parents with schizophrenia, bipolar disorder, and major depressive disorder: A meta-analysis of family high-risk studies. *Schizophrenia Bulletin, 40*(1), 28–38.

51 National Alliance on Mental Illness. (n.d.). *Anosognosia.* www.nami.org/About-Mental-Illness/Common-with-Mental-Illness/Anosognosia

52 Amador, X. F., Flaum, M., Andreasen, N. C., Strauss, D. H., Yale, S. A., Clark, S. C., & Gorman, J. M. (1994). Awareness of illness in schizophrenia and schizoaffective and mood disorders. *Archives of General Psychiatry, 51*(10), 826–836; Buckley, P. F., Wirshing, D. A., Bhushan, P., Pierre, J. M., Resnick, S. A., & Wirshing, W. C. (2007). Lack of insight in schizophrenia: impact on treatment adherence. *CNS Drugs, 21,* 129–141; Fennig, S., Everett, E., Bromet, E. J., Jandorf, L., Fennig, S. R., Tanenberg-Karant, M., & Craig, T. J. (1996). Insight in first-admission psychotic patients. *Schizophrenia Research, 22*(3), 257–263.

53 Amador, X. (2000). *I am not sick, I don't need help! How to help someone accept treatment.* Vida Press.

54 Substance Abuse and Mental Health Services Administration. (2021). *Key substance use and mental health indicators in the United States: Results from the 2020 National Survey on Drug Use and Health* (HHS Publication No. PEP21-07-01-003, NSDUH Series H-56).

55 Insel, T. (2022). *Healing: Our path from mental illness to mental health.* Penguin Press.

56 Deegan, P. E., Carpenter-Song, E., Drake, R. E., Naslund, J. A., Luciano, A., & Hutchison, S. L. (2017). Enhancing clients' communication regarding goals for using psychiatric medications. *Psychiatric Services, 68*(8), 771–775.

57 Zhang, M., Zhang, Y., & Kong, Y. (2019). Interaction between social pain and physical pain. *Brain Science Advances, 5*(4), 265–273.

58 Ringeisen, H., Edlund, M., Guyer, H., Geiger, P., Stambaugh, L., Dever, J., Liao, D., Carr, C., Peytchev, A., Reed, W., McDaniel, K., & Smith, T. (2023). *Mental and Substance Use Disorders Prevalence Study (MDPS): Findings Report*. RTI International.

59 Barbosa, C., Cowell, A. J., & Dowd, W. N. (2021). Alcohol consumption in response to the COVID-19 pandemic in the United States. *Journal of Addiction Medicine, 15*(4), 341–344.

60 Cartus, A. R., Li, Y., Macmadu, A., Goedel, W. C., Allen, B., Cerdá, M., & Marshall, B. D. (2022). Forecasted and observed drug overdose deaths in the US during the COVID-19 pandemic in 2020. *JAMA Network Open, 5*(3), e223418.

61 Substance Abuse and Mental Health Services Administration. (2021). *Key substance use and mental health indicators in the United States: Results from the 2020 National Survey on Drug Use and Health* (HHS Publication No. PEP21-07-01-003, NSDUH Series H-56). Center for Behavioral Health Statistics and Quality, Substance Abuse and Mental Health Services Administration

62 Bischof, G., Iwen, J., Freyer-Adam, J., & Rumpf, H. J. (2016). Efficacy of the Community Reinforcement and Family Training for concerned significant others of treatment-refusing individuals with alcohol dependence: A randomized controlled trial. *Drug and Alcohol Dependence, 163*, 179–185.

63 Meyers, R. J., Miller, W. R., Smith, J. E., & Tonigan, J. S. (2002). A randomized trial of two methods for engaging treatment-refusing drug users through concerned significant others. *Journal of Consulting and Clinical Psychology, 70*(5), 1182–1185.

64 American Psychiatric Association. (2022). *Diagnostic and statistical manual of mental disorders* (5th ed., Text Revision). Author.

65 Benjet, C., Bromet, E., Karam, E. G., Kessler, R. C., McLaughlin, K. A., Ruscio, A. M., Shahly, V., Stein, D., Petukhova, M., Hill, E., Alonso, J., Atwoli, L., Bunting, B., Bruffaerts, R., Caldas-de-Almeida, J., de Girolamo, G., Florescu, S., Gureje, O., Huang, Y.,. . . Koenen, K. C. (2016). Theepidemiology of traumatic event exposure worldwide: Results from the World Mental Health Survey Consortium. *Psychological Medicine, 46*(2), 327–343.

66 Grubaugh, A. L., Zinzow, H. M., Paul, L., Egede, L. E., & Frueh, B. C. (2011). Trauma exposure and posttraumatic stress disorder in adults with severe mental illness: A critical review. *Clinical Psychology Review, 31*(6), 883–899.

67 Goldstein, R. B., Smith, S. M., Chou, S. P., Saha, T. D., Jung, J., Zhang, H., Pickering, R., Ruan, W., Huang, B., & Grant, B. F. (2016). The epidemiology of DSM-5 posttraumatic stress disorder in the United States: Results from the National Epidemiologic Survey on Alcohol and Related Conditions-III. *Social Psychiatry and Psychiatric Epidemiology, 51*(8), 1137–1148.

68 Dallel, S., Cancel, A., & Fakra, E. (2018). Prevalence of posttraumatic stress disorder in schizophrenia spectrum disorders: A systematic review. *Neuropsychiatry, 8*(3), 1027–1037; Nabavi, B., Mitchell, A.J., & Nutt, D. (2015). A lifetime prevalence of comorbidity between bipolar affective disorder and anxiety disorders: A meta-analysis of 52 interview-based studies of psychiatric population. *EBioMedicine, 2*(10), 1405–1419.

69 Snicket, L. (2013). *When did you see her last? All the wrong questions, 2.* Little, Brown Books for Young Readers.

70 Tedeschi, R. G., Park, C. L., & Calhoun, L. G. (1998). *Posttraumatic growth: Positive changes in the aftermath of crisis.* Lawrence Erlbaum Associates, Publishers.

71 Centers for Disease Control and Prevention. Web-based Injury Statistics Query and Reporting System (WISQARS) Fatal Injury Reports. (2020, February 20). Retrieved September 4, 2022 from https:// webappa.cdc.gov/sasweb/ncipc/mortrate.html.

72 Ferrari, A. J., Norman, R. E., Freedman, G., Baxter, A. J., Pirkis, J. E., Harris, M. G., Page, A., Carnahan, E., Degenhardt, L, Vos, T., & Whiteford, H. A. (2014). The burden attributable to mental and substance use disorders as risk factors for suicide: Findings from the Global Burden of Disease Study 2010. *PloS One, 9*(4), e91936; Singhal, A., Ross, J., Seminog, O., Hawton, K., & Goldacre, M. J. (2014). Risk of self-harm and suicide in people with specific psychiatric and physical disorders: Comparisons between disorders using English national record linkage. *Journal of the Royal Society of Medicine, 107*(5), 194–204.

73 Glied, S., & Frank, R. G. (2014). Mental illness and violence: Lessons from the evidence. *American Journal of Public Health, 104*(2), e5–e6

74 Labrum, T., Solomon, P., & Marcus, S. (2020). Victimization and perpetration of violence involving persons with mood and other psychiatric disorders and their relatives. *Psychiatric Services, 71*(5), 498–501; Wang, L., Xu, J., Zou, H., Zhang, H., & Qu, Y. (2019). Violence against primary caregivers of people with severe mental illness and their knowledge and attitudes towards violence: A cross-sectional study in China. *Archives of Psychiatric Nursing, 33*(6), 167–176.

75 Labrum, T., Zingman, M. A., Nossel, I., & Dixon, L. (2021). Violence by persons with serious mental illness toward family caregivers and other relatives: A review. *Harvard Review of Psychiatry, 29*(1), 10–19; Peterson, J. K., Skeem, J., Kennealy, P., Bray, B., & Zvonkovic, A. (2014). How often and how consistently do symptoms directly precede criminal behavior among offenders with mental illness? *Law and Human Behavior, 38*(5), 439–449.

76 Linehan, M. M. (1993). *Cognitive-behavioral treatment of borderline personality disorder.* Guilford Press.

77 Desai, M. (2023, March 17). *The five things I wish I knew before becoming a family caregiver. Forbes.* www. forbes.com/sites/forbeseq/2023/03/17/the-five-things-i-wish-i-knew-before-becoming-a-family-caregiver/

78 Terlizzi, E.P., & Norris, T. (2021). *Mental health treatment among adults: United States, 2020.* Centers for Disease Control NCHS Data Brief No 419. www.cdc.gov/nchs/products/databriefs/db419.htm#section_4

79 Gloster, A. T., Walder, N., Levin, M. E., Twohig, M. P., & Karekla, M. (2020). The empirical status of acceptance and commitment therapy: A review of meta-analyses. *Journal of Contextual Behavioral Science, 18,* 181–192.

80 Fowler, D., Garety, P., & Kuipers, E. (1995). *Cognitive behaviour therapy for psychosis: Theory and practice.* John Wiley & Sons.

81 Frank, E. (2007). *Treating bipolar disorder: A clinician's guide to interpersonal and social rhythm therapy.* Guilford.

82 Beck, J. S. (2020). *Cognitive behavior therapy: Basics and beyond.* Guilford Publications.

83 Weissman, M. M., Markowitz, J. C., & Klerman, G. L. (2017). *The guide to interpersonal psychotherapy.* Updated and expanded edition. Oxford University Press.

84 Bond, G. R., Drake, R. E., & Becker, D. R. (2020). An update on individual placement and support. *World Psychiatry, 19*(3), 390–391.

85 McBain, R. K., Cantor, J., Pera, M. F., Breslau, J., Bravata, D. M., & Whaley, C. M. (2023). Mental health service utilization rates among commercially insured adults in the US during the first year of the COVID-19 pandemic. *JAMA Health Forum, 4*(1), e224936.

86 Kruse, C. S., Krowski, N., Rodriguez, B., Tran, L., Vela, J., & Brooks, M. (2017). Telehealth and patient satisfaction: A systematic review and narrative analysis. *BMJ Open, 7*(8), e016242.

87 Snoswell, C. L., Chelberg, G., De Guzman, K. R., Haydon, H. H., Thomas, E. E., Caffery, L. J., & Smith, A. C. (2021). The clinical effectiveness of telehealth: A systematic review of meta-analyses from 2010 to 2019. *Journal of Telemedicine and Telecare, 29*(9), 669–684; Varker, T., Brand, R. M., Ward, J., Terhaag, S., & Phelps, A. (2019). Efficacy of synchronous telepsychology interventions for people with anxiety, depression, posttraumatic stress disorder, and adjustment disorder: A rapid evidence assessment. *Psychological Services, 16*(4), 621–635.

88 Dixon, L. B., Goldman, H. H., Bennett, M. E., Wang, Y., McNamara, K. A., Mendon, S. J., Goldstein, A. B., Choi, C.-W.J., Lee, R. J., Lieberman, J. A. & Essock, S. M. (2015). Implementing coordinated specialty care for early psychosis: The RAISE Connection Program. *Psychiatric Services, 66*(7), 691–698; Lally, J., Ajnakina, O., Stubbs, B., Cullinane, M., Murphy, K. C., Gaughran, F., & Murray, R. M. (2017). Remission and recovery from first-episode psychosis in adults: Systematic review and meta-analysis of long-term outcome studies. *The British Journal of Psychiatry, 211*(6), 350–358; Read, H., & Kohrt, B. A. (2021). The history of coordinated specialty care for early intervention in psychosis in the United States: A review of effectiveness, implementation, and fidelity. *Community Mental Health Journal, 58,* 835–846.

INDEX

ABOUT THE AUTHORS

MICHELLE D. SHERMAN PHD ABPP (she/her) is a board-certified licensed clinical psychologist who has dedicated her career to supporting families dealing with a mental illness or history of trauma. She earned her PhD in clinical psychology from the University of Missouri–Columbia and then completed an internship at the University of Oklahoma Health Sciences Center. She went on to direct the Family Mental Health Program at the Oklahoma City VA Medical Center for 17 years and was a professor at the University of Oklahoma in the Department of Psychiatry and Behavioral Sciences. She then served as professor in the Department of Family Medicine and Community Health at the University of Minnesota Medical School. She recently transitioned to private practice in Minneapolis.

Dr. Sherman is a Fellow of the American Psychological Association (APA), and is board certified in Couple and Family Psychology. She is the Editor in Chief of *Couple and Family Psychology: Research and Practice*, the journal of APA's Society of Couple and Family Psychology. She was named the APA Family Psychologist of the Year (Society of Couple and Family Psychology) in 2022. She has published over 75 articles in peer-reviewed journals, has received over three million dollars in grant funding, and has given several hundred workshops nationally and internationally. She served on the Board of the Oklahoma National Alliance on Mental Illness (NAMI) for 14 years and now enjoys volunteering with the Minnesota NAMI affiliate.

DE ANNE SHERMAN (she/her), Michelle's mother, is a mental health advocate and educator. She graduated from St. Catherine University in St. Paul, Minnesota, with degrees in French, education, and speech and theater. She volunteers with NAMI-Minnesota, gives workshops with her daughter about mental illness in the family, and mentors people of all ages in the performing arts as a choreographer. DeAnne's mission is to affirm, educate, and empower others. She has strong passions for combatting stigma, offering hope to people who are hurting, celebrating diversity, and promoting open discussion about mental health.

The collaboration of psychologist and teacher, daughter and mother, brings true synergy to their work. The Shermans draw from their personal and professional life experiences which are the inspiration and foundation for their work.

Other books by Sherman and Sherman include: *I'm Not Alone: A Teen's Guide to Living with a Parent Who Has a Mental Illness; Finding My Way: A Teen's Guide to Living with a Parent Who Has Experienced Trauma;* **and** *My Story: Blogs by Four Military Teens* (**www.SeedsofHopeBooks.com**)